Residential Group Care in Community Context: Insights From the Israeli Experience

Zvi Eisikovits and Jerome Beker
Editors

The Haworth Press
New York • London

Residential Group Care in Community Context: Insights From the Israeli Experience has also been published as *Child & Youth Services,* Volume 7, Numbers 3/4, Summer 1985.

The Haworth Press, Inc., 28 East 22 Street, New York, NY 10010-6194
EUROSPAN/Haworth, 3 Henrietta Street, London WC2E 8LU England

Library of Congress Cataloging in Publication Data
Main entry under title:

Residential group care in community context.

   Published also as v. 7, no. 3/4 of Child & youth services.
   Includes bibliographies and index.
      1. Group homes for children—Israel. 2. Children—Institutional care—Israel. 3. Family policy—Israel. 4. Education—Israel. I. Eisikovits, Zvi. II. Beker, Jerome.
HV866.I75R47 1986   362.7'32'095694   85-7682
ISBN 0-86656-186-2

Residential Group Care in Community Context: Insights From the Israeli Experience

Child & Youth Services
Volume 7, Numbers 3/4

CONTENTS

III. POLICY IMPLICATIONS

IV. CONCLUSION

Introduction

Never the most popular intervention option for troubled children
and youth in the United States, Canada, and other western countries, residential group care has been particularly suspect in the past
decade. Much authoritative professional and lay opinion would have
us abandon it as an agent of positive and creative developmental
change in favor of non-institutional, community-based alternatives.
In this context, it seems appropriate to examine the "state of the
art" in a society, Israel's, that has enshrined group care over the
years as a powerfully effective approach not only in alleviating developmental deficits, but also in maximizing the contributions of its
most talented young people.

The winds of change have been felt in Israel as well, with
pressure toward establishing community linkages with residential
programs. But the group care tradition remains strong as the outcome of a powerful history described in the first article, by Anita
Weiner. Rivka Eisikovits follows up with an analysis of the constant
and complex interaction between Israeli culture and residential
group care, a perspective that should be instructive to those of us
who seek to understand the field elsewhere.

The placement process is presented by Zmira Laufer, with emphasis on the importance of the role of parents and whether placement is viewed as a stage in developmentally-oriented assistance to
the child and the family or as the objective of the intervention. Yitzhak Kashti and Mordecai Arieli then describe the internal dynamics
of residential group care centers and how they are changing in terms
that reflect life in the community as well, and Yochanan Wozner
follows with an analysis that accentuates the differences between the
two kinds of settings. In describing the community school movement in Israel, Ron Meier points to its possible role in bridging between residential settings and the home and community.

From somewhat contrasting perspectives emphasizing respectively the broader, societal influences and those more focused within
child and youth care systems, Nachman Sharon and Eliezer Jaffe examine public policy considerations related to residential care. Zvi
Eisikovits examines traditionally residential child and youth care

work as an occupation and a career, suggesting that adaptation is needed for it as well as the programs it serves to grow and adapt if both are to survive. In conclusion, the editors highlight major implications of the Israeli experience for child and youth care services elsewhere.

We hope this compendium will prove to be stimulating and useful to our colleagues in thinking about child and youth services in their own national contexts, and that it will contribute to the enhancement of programs and services for young people everywhere.

JB/ZE[1]

---

[1]The editors contributed equally in the editing of this issue. We wish to acknowledge the invaluable editorial and technical assistance provided by Margaret Atkinson, Emily Beker, and Edna Guttmann.

I.
Historical and Social Context

Institutionalizing Institutionalization: The Historical Roots of Residential Care in Israel

Anita Weiner

ABSTRACT. The pattern of group care in Israel today has its ideological and pragmatic roots in the pre-State, Mandate period. The utopian exuberance of the 1920s led to the creation of model "children's villages" which later expanded rapidly to meet the crisis demands of the 1930s and 1940s. A process of mass institutionalization and bureaucratic inflexibility gradually took over, but the ideological commitment to collective group care has remained central in Israeli child welfare services.

The purpose of this article is to examine the historical processes which led to the institutionalization of residential care for children and youth in the Jewish community Israel. These processes were born of historical imperative and ideological fervor and their convergence has been a powerful one. They began over fifty years ago, and they continue to impact the field of residential care in Israel today.

THE HISTORICAL IMPERATIVE

It is not within the purpose of this article to chronicle the dramatic events which nearly annihilated the Jewish population of Europe during the 1930s and 1940s. Suffice it to say that due to the Holocaust, thousands of children without families sought refuge in Israel prior to the establishment of the State in 1948. They were in urgent need of shelter and care, and dozens of residential facilities (over 150 by 1945) were created to meet the need.

Anita Weiner, School of Social Work, University of Haifa, Mount Carmel, Haifa 31 999, Israel.

Although the urgency of the need was the major impetus for the original establishment of the institutions, the fact that Israel has consistently had one of the world's highest percentage of children and youth living in residential care for the past 35 years cannot be explained on pragmatic grounds alone. It was the power of ideological commitment which turned the shelters of the 1940s into a deeply rooted social movement. Created out of necessity, they became a way of life. Some major ideological dilemmas for those responsible for institutional programs in the pre-State period resulted.

1. Planned Utopia vs. Flexible Intervention

The ideological roots of residential care in Israel are largely Utopian in origin. With the optimism of the 1920s following the Balfour Declaration and its promise of Jewish Statehood, educators were determined to create ideal residential environments for the socialization of the new, young pioneer. These educators felt that residential care should reflect the Utopian ideals of the society, and their children and youth should adapt themselves to environments planned for them so they could become better citizens. They made the assumption that the needs of the individual and of the family should be subordinated to those of the group. Kellner (1974) calls this approach to social planning the Platonic approach.

Other educators, such as Eder, Szold, Idelson, and Berger, advocated a different, more flexible and humanistic approach. Their assumption was that there is no ideal residential environment for the socialization of children, and that the institutions of society must serve the needs of the individual. Residential services should be flexible, offering a wide variety of alternative solutions to children in distress. Kellner calls this the Maimonidean approach. The advocates of this second view were in the minority during the early, critical years, and the Platonic, utopian approach continues to influence residential care workers in Israel to this day.

2. Collective vs. Family Child-Rearing

The idea of the collective settlement (such as the kibbutz) was born early in the century. To many of the young pioneers who came from Europe to participate in the creation of a new society, group support and the organization of collective labor replaced the extended family and eased the loneliness resulting from severed ties. By the early 1920s, children growing up in the collective settlements were living in communal childrens' homes, and the question of collective versus family education for the socialization of children became a widely debated educational issue. Talmon (1970) claims that the advocacy of collective group care was a reflection of the need to make a "radical separation from the past." "Cut off from the support of family ties, the young pioneers tended to transfer the main responsibility for the socialization of their children from parents to society."

Less than five percent of the population lived in the collective settlements, but the impact of their ideological outlook far outweighed their proportional representation. The key issue became whether collective group care was a preferable environment for child-rearing in the new society. Much residential care in Israel continues to reflect the view that it is.

3. Rural vs. Urban Child Rearing

During the pre-State period, urban environments were generally considered to be unsuitable for the proper socialization of pioneer youth. Rural, agricultural settings were selected as the appropriate environment for residential care. In such a setting the "corrupting" influence of the big city could be counteracted, and the children could be exposed to the values of collective agricultural labor (Cohen, 1970).

Since the majority of the Jewish population in Israel was always urban, the removal of children and youth to remote agricultural residential facilities contained an implied rejection of family ties. The romanticization of rural life also reinforced the transfer of responsibility for child-rearing from the immediate family (the urban family) to society at large (the rural agricultural residential facility), another theme that continues to influence residential programs today.

4. Religious vs. Secular Socialization

During the pre-State period, there was no compulsory education law and an intricate network of Hebrew education for the many sectors of the Jewish population was organized by the community. The issue of religious vs. secular schooling was heatedly debated, and ultimately four separate school systems were created. Two were religious (one "modern," the other, ultratraditional) and two were secular (General Zionists and Labor). Residential institutions for children were each linked to one of these school systems, and child welfare workers had to take into account the religious/political background of a child when making a placement decision. This problem was more complex than would at first appear, since the places available often did not match the children in need of placement. When the two ideological elements of collective socialization and rural environment were added to the religious issue, the problems multiplied.

During the pre-State years, there were very few religious agricultural collectives, and those could absorb only a small proportion of the religious children in need of placement. The situation became even more acute after 1934, with the arrival of Youth Aliyah groups from Germany and Austria. An agreement had been made with the Jewish community in Germany that twenty five percent of the youth arriving in Israel would be from religious homes. However, after the first group of 25 religious youth were absorbed in Kibbutz Yavneh, no more religious collective rural facilities were available, and it became urgent to set up religious residential facilities for the hundreds of religious children and youth continuing to arrive.

In 1943, 716 orphaned children who had miraculously escaped from Poland arrived in Israel via Teheran (they were called the "Children of Teheran"). An immediate clamor arose among the competing secular and religious movements, all of whom were eager to adopt and socialize these orphaned children. In this case as in many others, Henrietta Szold, widely viewed as the founder of modern residential care in Israel, was in charge of residential care for the orphans; her flexible, individualistic approach did not find favor in the eyes of the competing religious and secular groups. She went to great lengths to safeguard the personal tendencies of the children in the face of conflicting political and ideological pressures from the various religious and secular pressure groups. They saw it as their mission to "capture" these vulnerable orphans and to socialize them in their own residences—thus, the stakes were high. Szold arranged to have each child interviewed individually to identify their preferences and family backgrounds to be considered. The representatives of the competing educational ideologies did not trust one another, however, and they insisted that each be represented at the individual interviews, so the children had to state their preferences in front of a panel (Erlich, 1946; Lowenthal, 1942; Zeitlin,

1952). This is a dramatic example of the degree of conflict that existed among groups of religious and secular child care educators, and it, too, is a continuing tension in the residential care field. In sum, predetermined vs. flexible intervention, collective vs. family child-rearing, rural vs. urban socialization, and religious vs. secular education were the significant issues of conflict among child care workers. As attempts were made to resolve these conflicting issues, an ideological spectrum of child care in Israel emerged. Most of the residential facilities created during the Mandate period fell within at least one of the categories in this spectrum. Each of these categories will now be analyzed in greater depth.

A SPECTRUM OF IDEOLOGICAL APPROACHES TO RESIDENTIAL CARE

Point One: Immediate Short-term Aid with Family Continuity
Point Two: Environmental Change and "Social Therapy"
Point Three: The Individual in a Group Setting
Point Four: Manual Labor and the Educational Group
Point Five: The Youth Collective and the New Pioneer

Point One:Immediate Short-Term Aid with Family Continuity

During the Mandate period, there was only one significant educator who systematically supported the approach of family continuity and community contact (Weiner, 1979). This was Dr. Montigue David Eder (1866-1936), a student of Freud and a British psychoanalyst. He arrived in Palestine in 1918 and was placed in charge of rescue operation for victims of World War One.

Eder had strong objections to the establishment of large, closed institutions to house the thousands of orphaned children he found in the country, for whom rapid, universal solutions were required. Instead, he created the Palestine Orphan Committee (POC), which devised an elaborate system of foster care within the various Jewish communities in the country. He believed that children raised in large residential facilities are handicapped in their contacts with the "real world." "The boundaries of their existence are very narrow, the large world outside with its variety and abundance never gets to them. The younger the children are when they arrive at such a place, and the more thoroughly they are supervised, the more their world will be ruined when they leave the place'' (Eder, 1919-1924). During the ten years of its activity (1918-1928), the POC was true to Eder's principles and cared for the 4,000 children under its jurisdiction according to his approach. Continuity was maintained with the remnants of each child's family, and children were visited by POC child care workers on a bi-monthly basis. Reports were filed regularly on foster home conditions, and weekly accounts were received from the children's schools about illnesses and school absences.

Twelve small residential homes were established for those children for whom no foster homes were found and all twelve homes were closed as scheduled when the residents reached independence and had learned occupations which enabled them to be self-supporting. Eder was deeply opposed to perpetuating institutions that had already successfully fulfilled their original goals, and the residences he established were the only ones deliberately closed according to plan in all the decades to follow.

In light of current thinking, Eder's plan of intervention can be viewed as a sound one and could serve as a basis for treatment planning even today. However, due to the strong impact of ideological commitment, his approach was almost immediately forgotten and remained largely unacknowledged during the remainder of the Mandate period. In a 1936 report of the Social Welfare Department, it was even stated that foster care had never been attempted or heard of by the local Jewish population (National Committee for the . . . , 1936). It was not until the 1960s that the Archives of the Palestine Orphan Committee were reviewed, and the early history of foster care, and short term intervention for the maintenance of family continuity was acknowledged as a legitimate part of Israel's child care history.

Point Two:Environmental Change and "Social Therapy"

The second approach on the ideological spectrum was an approach which advocated child placement as a concrete expression of social justice. An assumption was made that children should be reared in "suitable" homes which reflect the dominant norms of the society. If an authorized source of authority diagnosed a home as "unsuitable," the intervention of choice was the removal of the child to a better environment. It was an approach which relied on environmental change and was called "Sociale Therapie" by its advocates, the majority of whom were social workers (Wronsky, 1924).

Social work, which began to develop as a profession at the turn of the century, was vulnerable to this "moral authoritarianism" due to the early preponderance of middle class volunteers with unquestioned values determined by their social class. The Institute of Training for Social Workers, which opened in Berlin in 1908 under the direction of Alice Solomon, was an early example of the "moral authoritarian," social therapy approach. It was in this Institute that most of the social workers who immigrated to Israel in the 1930s were trained, and its theoretical approach had great impact on the early years of residential care for children in Israel.

The Social Therapy approach favored a socialist society with humanitarian values, which strived to improve the conditions of the underprivileged. The role of the social worker was mainly to serve as a diagnostician who determined whether a given home environment was a suitable one for the rearing of a good future citizen, obviously a process particularly prone to the imposition of the worker's own values. The act of social therapy came into play when a child was removed from a residential environment found unsuitable, and placed in one considered more conducive to his proper development.

The social therapy approach did not oppose parental education or the rearing of children in families. It did, however, provide a wide margin for the moral judgement of individual workers. In an environment which idealized residential care, social workers with a social therapy approach were particularly vulnerable. By contrast, the professional literature of the 1930s in child care abounded with statements concerning the importance of the family and the need for society to provide for weak families. In practice, however, largely due to the pressures just cited, family treatment generally consisted of diagnosis followed by residential placement.

In addition to the impact of the Berlin Social Work Institute, there was another factor which had significant influence on residential care in Israel. It had been the policy of the Berlin Institute to accept only people with experience, those who had previously been engaged in community work. Most social workers from the Berlin Institute who immigrated to Israel in the 1930s had worked, prior to their studies, in one of the institutions for dependent children in Europe. Their work in these institutions geared them toward the acceptance of residential care as a natural, acceptable option. With their immigration to Israel, child placement as social therapy received a significant push forward. When the Child Placement Center was established by Wronsky, a former lecturer at the Berlin Institute in Tel-Aviv in 1934, the number of children referred for residential care among both immigrant and native-born families rose significantly.

Point Three:The Individual in a Group Setting

A third approach evident in the early establishment of residential facilities was based on the belief that group care is a useful background for individual rehabilitation. Three European educators active during this period, were particularly influential—August Aichorn, Janos Korczak and Martin Buber.

Aichorn (1935), an influential psychoanalyst concerned with group care, opened a small institution for the rehabilitation of delinquents in Germany in the 1920s. His account of work done there had a strong influence on David Idelson, director of the Tel-Aviv Municipality youth department during the Mandate period, who established a small institution for delinquents from slum neighborhoods in 1934. In Idelson's institute, as in Aichorn's, the group served mainly as a backdrop for youth in treatment; the focus of the work was on the development of a one-to-one relationship. It was through this relationship that the youth was directed toward rehabilitation.

Idelson also took a summer course taught by Ziegfried Berfeld in Vienna and visited the children's villages of Shatzky and Makarenko in Russia. He rejected the Russians' extreme collective approach, and most of his activities were directed towards the individual, with emphasis on inner change. Under Idelson's influence, the residential institutions for children founded by the Tel-Aviv Municipality were small, maintained an individualized approach, and supported community and urban contacts (Idelson, 1956).

Another group care educator with an individualistic approach was Janos Korczak (1967). Korczak, born in Poland in 1878, was a pediatrician and author of children's books. He established two orphanages for Jewish children and developed a special approach that encouraged self-government, and the children's sense of responsibility for themselves and society. His approach was unostentatious, dedicated, and pragmatic. Both of the institutions he founded were located within urban areas, and there was no attempt to isolate them from the surrounding community. The rules of the institutions, e.g., on work, food, and dress, paralleled the norms of life outside, so as to accustom the children to the realities of life. Children who worked were paid for their efforts; and children who took better care of their clothes received better clothes. Korczak also wrote educational books for parents and tended to encourage family contact for those children who had families. Korczak visited Israel twice before World War Two, and he apparently considered transferring his institutions to Israel. Both institutions were destroyed by the Nazis, and Korczak died a martyr's death in 1942 together with the children. His influence was felt by many child care workers in pre-State Israel.

In addition to the ideas of Aichorn and Korczak, Martin Buber's philosophical approach to education had an impact on early residential care in Israel. Although Buber himself did not establish any institutions for children, his impact was felt through his commitment to the Jewish tradition and its sources and through his opposition to political affiliations in education. His "I-Thou" approach (Buber, 1958) implicitly rejected the collectivization of education. Among the European educators influenced by Buber who came to Israel and established residential institutions for children was Beate Berger, the director of "Ahava."

Berger was the director of an institution for Jewish refugee children in Berlin. The institution had a traditionally religious and Zionist educational approach. Community contacts were maintained, and ties with the children's families were encouraged. With the rise of Hitler, Berger transferred the entire institution to Haifa, Israel, in 1934, as part of the Youth Aliyah movement. Despite the pressure for political and religious affiliation, Berger maintained her commitment to the observance of Jewish tradition without either orthodox religious affiliation or other political, ideological commitments. Her commitment was to an individualistic approach within a group setting.

Point Four:Manual Labor and the Educational Group

The sacredness of manual labor was the central idea held by two major educators who had a great influence on pre-State residential care in Israel: A. D. Gordon and Pestolozzi.

A. D. Gordon (1856-1921) was a firm believer in the value of physical labor. Beginning in 1904, he worked as an agricultural laborer on a Jewish settlement in pre-Mandate Palestine. He believed that only a return to the land to manual labor could rehabilitate the Jewish people, and he served as a personal example until his death. Gordon believed that change in a nation must come about through an internal change of values within each individual. He was opposed to social planning and group education, since he felt that educators with strong personalities tend to force their opinion on those being educated (Gordon, 1952).

Gordon's belief in manual labor was widely respected and accepted, and the principle of labor became a recurring theme in education and in residential care. Thus, socialization of the new, idealistic pioneer continued to be associated with manual labor and working the land. On the other hand, Gordon's vehement opposition to group education was ignored. Educators with "strong personalities" took up the banner of manual labor and applied it enthusiastically in group education. Even today, Gordon's views on social planning are far less known than his belief in the importance of working the land.

Pestolozzi's (1746-1827) approach, in contrast to Gordon's, emphasized both labor and the group. Pestolozzi established an agricultural institution in Switzerland for abandoned orphans. Based on his writings, Kershensteiner, a German educator (1865-1932) created the concept of the "School of Labor." Kershensteimer's books were translated into Hebrew and were widely read by child care workers in Israel throughout the Mandate period. These books emphasized the importance of work, education, and group activities in the shaping of a child's personality (Kershensteiner, 1929, 1939).

It was Bernfeld (1892-1953), however, who was the first European Jewish educator to combine the principle of labor, group education, and the Zionist ideal. He established a Jewish orphanage in Vienna in 1919 and published his educational principles in a book (Bernfeld, 1919) that had a long term impact. During the 1920s, educators and child care workers came from Israel to attend his summer courses. He advocated the founding of "children's villages" in Israel to provide pioneer training for both native born and immigrant children.

The first educator to establish such a "childrens' village" in Israel was Moshe Kalvary. He was an enthusiastic follower of both Bernfeld and Buber, and he immigrated to Israel in 1923. Eder, who opposed children's institutions, had just left the country, and Kalvary succeeded in convincing the POC to enable him to fulfill his dream of establishing a rural agricultural, educational institution. "Meir Schefeya" was opened in August 1923 with 60 orphaned girls who were to be instilled with a love of labor, a love of society, and a commitment to the Jewish traditions (Kalvary, 1924).

The second educator to establish a "children's village" according to the ideals of Bernfeld and Buber was Ziegfried Lehman (1892-1958). Lehman, a physician and educator, founded a Jewish orphanage in Kovno after World War One and immigrated to Ben Shemen, Israel, in 1927 together with its staff and children. During the remainder of the Mandate period, "Ben Shemen" absorbed both native-born and immigrant children from Youth Aliyah, a worldwide organization to foster the immigration of needy Jewish children to Israel.

Lehman's educational approach at Ben Shemen was based on four principles: Working the land; Self-government of the children (community life); Education towards peace and understanding between nations; and Education in Jewish traditions. Ben Shemen was not affiliated with any political or religious party, and Lehman encouraged the children to choose between the various youth movements. Although Lehman did not oppose family ties, the geographical isolation of the institution and its rural agricultural character did not encourage easy access to families or to community ties. Ben Shemen was the largest residential institution in the country during the Mandate period, working with up to 650 children. It has a profound impact on child care workers throughout the country, many of whom had either worked, visited, or had been educated there.

Point Five:The Youth Collective and the New Pioneer

The final component of the spectrum is the approach of the "youth collective" as a total youth community. The difference between a social group and a youth community is that "the social group usually aims at a limited content of educational aid, while the youth community (aims at) a general education of the young person in his entirety, at all his necessary educational needs" (Ron-Polanyi, 1964).

Makarenko and Schtazky from Russia and Wyniken from Germany were the main idealogues of this approach. They believed that only through the complete severance of ties between the child and his family could a child's previous patterns of thought and behavior be changed and a "new person" made out of him. Makarenko

(1954) described his work with street gangs in Russia, whose members, under his guidance turned into constructive citizens with positive attitudes. Makarenko attributes this change to the fact that the young people became dependent on the judgment of the group and learned to behave in accordance with the group's demands. This was achieved through the rather extreme measure of banning individual conversations, which were seen as fostering self-pity. Instead, every problem, large or small was to be the topic of a group discussion between the members of the children's society (Makarenko, 1954).

In Israel, the cutting of ties between most of the young pioneers and their families in the diaspora and the necessity for creating a new society formed an environment in which the idea of the youth collective had particular appeal. Many child care workers felt that the children in their care required a complete re-education and that family ties should consequently, be discouraged.

Wyniken's (1931) attitude towards the parental role in this respect was also a negative one. He saw collective education as a healthy substitute for "the sentimental worship of the individual personality." Wyniken claimed that "education is, in a more defined sense, the inclusion of the individual's will into the social will." He believed that, "In most cases the family lacks the necessary moral level for education in purity and objectivity." He advocated the total severance of contact between children and parents and was against the "worshipping of personality." Only thus could a new, healthy generation be educated. Family ties led to too much coddling and prevented the child from coping on his own. Jewish families were, in his opinion, famous for too much coddling. This strong ideological orientation fell on fertile soil in Israel. It was a period of acute social stress, when family life was being forcibly ruptured, and the opportunity to combine an ideological justification for these disruptions with a vision of the creation of an ideal new society was irresistible.

In 1934, with the establishment of Youth Aliyah, the integration of the national Zionist movement and the dream of the youth collective reached its climax. Recha Freier, the founder of Youth Aliyah, had been the first to suggest sending Zionist youth from Europe to existing agricultural collectives in Israel. It was believed that "by bringing children to Israel, and away from their families, they were being made members of a larger family which is the nation" (Bentwich, 1944). As tens, then hundreds, and then thousands of children arrived in Israel from war-threatened Europe, they were sent to newly established youth homes in the collective settlements. When the capacity of these settlements to absorb new groups came to an end—for religious children, this was almost immediately—the establishment of new residential facilities became imperative.

An acute issue in the founding of these new group care facilities was the tendency of politically minded educators to take advantage of vulnerable orphans in order to apply their doctrines. These educators tended to believe in the "youth collective," and to be followers of Makarenko and Wyniken. Thus, many refugee orphans arriving during World War Two, regardless of background or individual preference, found themselves placed in politically-oriented collective group care facilities. As these facilities multiplied, children born in Israel also became candidates. Freier arrived in Israel in 1941 and immediately advocated the collective, rural socialization of children born in Israel's slums. The residential facilities in Israel had by then become the primary vehicle of political and ideological indoctrination of Israel's youth population.

THE PROCESS OF INSTITUTIONALIZING INSTITUTIONALIZATION

These ideologies of child rearing struck deep chords of sympathy within the Jewish community. During the early Mandate years, educators spoke to the heart of the small and struggling Jewish community, and a belief in the group care of children was seeded and took root. New and experimental childrens' villages were established and admired, and an atmosphere of hope and of conviction was prevalent.

However, as the emergency pressures from the impending Holocaust of European Jewry and the Middle East increased in the 1930s, a sense of urgency began to take precedence. Saving lives became the first priority, and it was necessary to find immediate, practical solutions for the refugee children arriving unpredictably, but in ever-increasing numbers.

Since several experimental children's villages had already been established, the most efficient approach was to expand those already in existence and to set up new ones on the same model. The whole ideological movement was forced to shift gears, and the order of the day became systematization and an almost routine sense of urgency. There was no viable alternative to collective group care, and the "era of efficiency" had begun. For the next twenty years, child care workers expended great energy and ingenuity on expanding the network of residential institutions, which led to increasing bureaucratization. This process of institutionalization was in full swing during the 1940s and 1950s. Two major expressions of this shift were the Child Placement Center and the development of physical facilities.

The Child Placement Center

After the establishment of the Social Welfare Ministry in 1932 with its tens of local welfare offices, it became apparent that a fierce competition was developing among the local offices for residential placement contacts. Social workers sought personal links to institutional directors, to help guarantee that they could find places for the local children in their charge. A system of coordination was needed, and Wronsky was put in charge of a Child Placement Center which began operations in March 1934.

A formalized referral system was established and, as soon as a place became available in a residential facility or a new residence was founded, all the local offices were informed. During its first years, 450 children were registered. Three years later, the number rose to 1,350. These increasing numbers, in turn, created pressures toward the expansion of existing residential facilities and the establishment of new ones.

Land, Buildings, and Budgets

The second expression of the growing process of formalization or bureaucratization can be rather graphically documented through the authorization of public land and buildings. Throughout the Mandate period, there was constant pressure on the Jewish National Council to allocate funds for the building and expansion of residential institutions. During the years 1935-1945, Youth Aliyah, according to general belief, placed most of its immigrant youth in established agricultural settlements. In actual fact, however, Youth Aliyah allocated 96,376 Palestinian Pounds for the building of institutions and youth homes (Youth Aliyah, 1944-1945). This was an astronomical sum of money in those days. In order to grasp the vastness of this sum, suffice it to say that the monthly cost of upkeep for a child per month was between one and a half to five Palestinian Pounds!

The story of "Ahuzat Yeladim," an institution on Mt. Carmel, is a classic example of the process of institutionalization. Having begun operations in 1932 as a summer camp on land donated by a Haifa businessman, it had by the next year extended its "summer season" and the number of children accommodated from around the country had been increased from 50 to 100. In 1943 when a European refugee boat (The Patria) was sunk by the British off the coast of Haifa, over 100 children were rescued and interred by the British Army at a camp in Atlit. Henrietta Szold worked tirelessly for the release of the children and, when she succeeded, they were brought to Ahuzat Yeladim, which was immediately made into a permanent residence and has, for the last forty years, housed 120 children yearly.

Permanent institutions entail staff and physical upkeep, which require predictable, continuing financial support. The process of institutionalization found its way into the various budgetary allocations of the Jewish community during the Mandate period. During the 1920s, before the establishment of the Welfare Department, assistance for children had been based upon a spontaneous response to national calamity. With the establishment of an official Welfare Department, the flexibility (yet unreliability) of the previous system was replaced by a more reliable but relatively inflexible one.

In order to ensure that sufficient funds would be available to cover the expenses of the residential facilities, the decision was made that costs of residential care would be covered by the National Welfare budget, rather than through the local offices. Since local welfare offices have, notoriously tended to be short of funds throughout the history of organized welfare, this bureaucratic decision, made in December, 1934, had immediate repercussions. It provided a financial incentive that matched the deeply felt group care ideology and the enthusiastic response was reflected in the National Welfare Budget. In 1935, close to 40 percent of the Jewish community's welfare budget was allocated to the funding of children's residential institutions. By June of 1940, the percentage rose to 60 percent, and it never went below 50 percent in the pre-Statehood period.

A cycle had been established whereby the institutions which were constantly being created were dependent on ever-increasing budgets to justify their existence, and on ever increasing numbers of children to justify their budgetary expenditures.

SUMMARY

It has been the purpose of this article to analyze the historical and ideological roots of residential group care in Israel. Due to the dramatic events of the 1930s and 1940, the ideological seeds that had been sown in the previous decade for the development of utopian childrens' villages gave way to needed pragmatic solutions to large scale distress and child welfare crises. In founding these villages, prominent educators had set out to mold the new Israeli pioneer, who would be exposed to rural, agricultural labor and to the socialization of a youth collective but, as these goals were necessarily compromised, a process of institutionalization took precedence. The growing bureaucracy developed a momentum of its own, which was further reinforced by the continuing ideological input. These two forces, the ideological and the bureaucratic, continue to influence all aspects of residential group care in Israel today.

REFERENCES

Aichorn, A. (1935). *Wayward youth.* New York: Viking Press.
Bentwich, N. (1944). *Jewish youth come home.* London: Victor Gollancz Ltd.
Bernfeld, Z. (1919). The nation and youth. Merchavia, Sifriyat Hapoalim, republished 1948 (both in Hebrew).
Buber, M. (1958). *I and thou.* New York: Charles Scribner's Sons.
Cohen, E. (1970). *The city in Zionist ideology.* Jerusalem: Urban Studies Institute, Eliezer Kaplan School of Economics and Social Sciences.
Eder, M. D. (1919). Supervision of orphans. *Education.* Jaffa (in Hebrew).
Erlich, E. (1946). *Fighting angel: The story of Henrietta Szold.* New York: Behrman House.
Gordon, A. D. (1952). *The nation and labour.* Jerusalem: HaHistradut Hatzionit.
Idelson, D. (1956). *Youth in danger.* Merchavia, Sifriyat Hapoalim, Hakibbutz Haartzi (in Hebrew).
Kalvary, M. (1924). The rural orphanage for girls in Meir Schefaya. *Education.* Tel Aviv (in Hebrew).
Kellner, J. (1974). Contrasting models of community welfare: Plato and Maimonides. *Journal of Jewish Communal Services, 51*(1), 67-72.
Kershensteiner, G. (1929). *Concept and character education.* Jerusalem: Otzar HaMoreh (in Hebrew).
Kershensteiner, G. (1939). The school of labor. Jerusalem: *Educational Echo* (in Hebrew).
Korczak, J. (1967). *Selected works of Janusz Korczak.* Warsaw: Scientific Publications Foreign Cooperation Center of the Central Institute for Scientific, Technical and Economic Information.

Lowenthal, M. (1942). *Henrietta Szold: Life and letters.* New York: Viking Press.

Makarenko, A. S. (1954). *A book for parents.* Moscow: Foreign Languages Publishing House.

The National Committee for the Community of Israel. (1936). *News about social work in the land of Israel.* Bulletin. Jerusalem: Ministry of Social Welfare (in Hebrew).

Ron-Polanyi, Y. (1964). *The youth collective in Israel, what is it?* Tel Aviv: Ihud Hakevutzot VeHakibbutzim, Education Department (in Hebrew).

Talmon-Garber, Y. (1970). *The individual and society on the kibbutz.* Jerusalem: Hebrew University Press (in Hebrew).

Weiner, A. (1979). *Differential trends in child placement in the land of Israel 1918-1945.* Unpublished doctoral dissertation, Hebrew University, Jerusalem.

Wronsky, S. (1924). *Sociale therapie.* Berlin: Private printing (in German).

Wyniken, G. (1931). School and the youth culture. In M. Adler (Ed.), *The men of tomorrow: Ideas for socialistic education* (p. 42). Warsaw: The Central Guard Cooperative (in German).

Youth Aliyah Financial Report. (1944-1945). Jerusalem: Youth Aliyah Financial Archives (in Hebrew).

Zeitlin, R. (1952). *Henrietta Szold: Record of life.* New York: The Dial Press.

Children's Institutions in Israel as Mirrors of Social and Cultural Change

Rivka A. Eisikovits

ABSTRACT. The study of any major social institution yields insight into macro-social processes. Emerging trends in the social function of children's institutions in Israel can be analyzed fruitfully from this perspective, since close to twenty percent of the youth are educated in residential settings. Such a study is expected to enhance our understanding of the normative culture. The use to which a society puts its institutions for children and youth is a good measure of long range national goals.

In his article, "The State System, Schooling and Cognitive and Motivational Patterns," Cohen (1975) maintains that:

> The analysis of the development of specific social institutions depends on the premise that social forms can only emerge, flourish and be sustained in sociocultural atmospheres that are conducive to them. Each of these social forms must be regarded as an aspect of a population's adaption to its total environment. (p. 103)

Thus the study of any major social institution yields insight into macro-social processes. Emerging trends in the social function of children's institutions in Israel can be analyzed fruitfully from this perspective, since close to twenty percent of the youth are educated in residential settings (Kashti, Arieli, & Wozner, 1981). Such a study can hopefully enhance our understanding of the normative culture in Israel; the use to which a society puts its institutions for children and youth is a good measure of long range national goals.

Rivka A. Eisikovits, School of Education and School of Social Work, University of Haifa, Mount Carmel, Haifa, 31 999, Israel.

Cohen also maintains that, while:

> Man may affect the character of the institutions he creates, their emergency in the first place, or their loss, are not matters of deliberate social policy. (p. 109)

However, it should be borne in mind when studying such educational institutions that, if their "character" at any given period is out of touch with the needs of the society, this in itself can bring about their "loss" or disappearance. Hence in an indirect way man *does* control the very existence of his culture's basic social institutions—a less deterministic stance than the one put forth by Cohen. This, then, is another premise in the light of which the role of residential education in Israel will be assessed.

Day schools in most western democracies define their central goal as primarily one of training the mind, teaching subject matter, and are only minimally preoccupied with moral or ideological training. Thus residential education has advantages over day schooling when one or several of the following objectives prevail:

1. When character formation is the major goal of formal education.
2. When the need for a total and supervised ideological immersion of the young is of primary national interest.

Some years ago Wallace (1961) compared the relative role allocated to primary and secondary socializing agencies under a variety of political regimes. In revolutionary societies, he contended, the state claims as close to complete control as possible over the whole child at the expense of minimizing the child-caring role of the family, considered a suspect, even subversive institution. In this framework, residential educational settings have obvious advantages over day schools.

In the U.S.S.R., for example, a high percentage of children are educated in boarding schools (Bronfenbrenner, 1970; King, 1974; Weeks, 1974). During the pre-statehood period in Israel, the pressure of creating a new state with the highly normative idealistic orientation which characterized that period, and the consequences of the Holocaust which left many orphans in need of care (Wolins, 1971), made residential schools a rather adaptive educational alternative. In the U.S., on the other hand, where individualism and self-determination have traditionally been focal educational values, boarding schools have tended to be viewed as a more suitable instructional vehicle for "problematic" rather than normal children.[1]

3. When the end goal is defined as education for membership in a socially elite group such as, in the ironically named "public schools" of Britain (King, 1974), the formation of a "gentleman."

In all these cases it is assumed that closer attention to a holistic educational experience can be paid in the more fully supervised residential environment.

"The essence of schooling is that it serves the adoption of universalistic values, criteria and standards of performance" (Cohen, 1975, p. 113). This paper argues that only as long as a parity between universalitic and particularistic (subgroup) values prevails is a coherence between goals and means maintained. The residential school both reflects and attempts to respond to larger social needs, thereby serving as an effective socializatory vehicle.

THE PRE-STATEHOOD PERIOD

Detailed descriptions and analyses of the variety of residential educational institutions in either the pre- or the post-statehood period in Israel have already been done (Kashti, 1979; Kashti, Arieli, Wozner, 1981; Wolins and Gottesman, 1971). Residential schools existed ever since the beginning of the Zionist settlement. Some functioned as an integral part of various kibbutzim. Others were operated as organizationally autonomous entities, such as agricultural boarding schools or youth villages that attempted to recreate and instill in their students the same pioneering spirit that the kibbutz came to symbolize. These schools served several categories of students: the offspring of rural Jewish settlers and urban Zionists, new immigrant youth who had received a preparatory Zionist and agricultural education in their countries of origin prior to their ar-

---

1. Wolins (1974) claims that this orientation is gradually changing. His research has dispelled the myth of the detrimental impact of institutional life on normal child development (Bowlby, 1952) by demonstrating that well adjusted children live in group arrangements such as the Israeli kibbutz, the Soviet boarding school, the Austrian "kindersdorf," etc. The increasing need for out-of-home child care as a result of the dramatically rising trend of maternal employment has been another influential factor.

rival, and refugee children from the Nazi Holocaust who were brought to Israel by Youth Aliyah to start a new life (Kashti, Arieli, and Wozner, 1981; Wolins, 1971).

Under such conditions, maximal correspondence between universalistic and particularistic educational goals could be assured and the residential schools proved to be optimally adapted to the needs of the society they served. Wolins has put this equation rather succinctly in the context of educating Youth Aliyah's charges (Wolins and Gottesman, 1971, p. 5):

> Absorption meant preparation for membership in a kibbutz and for citizenship in the country. It meant the acceptance of an egalitarian, collectivist ideology, a life of labor on the land, self-fulfillment through group and even national accomplishment.

THE POST-STATEHOOD SCENE

After the achievement of statehood this balance was gradually upset. The breaking point occurred when the government set up a state-supported educational system providing universal free schooling. The initial revolutionary pioneering fervor was replaced increasingly by an "established" social climate. According to Wallace's (1961) theory mentioned earlier, in more conservative societies, the importance of schools as central socializing media gradually declines as the individual family group gains in social credibility and comes to be regarded as a "loyal" or "trustworthy" agent of primary socialization. In Israeli society, the indisputable advantages of the residential school for the earlier period are decreasingly apparent now.

A rapid trend towards urbanization took place in the fifties, and with it a shift in value orientation from egalitarianism to individualism (Eisenstadt, 1967; Kleinberger, 1969). In an increasingly meritocratic system, credentials were increasingly emphasized as a means of upward mobility. Within this new context formal education grew in importance and partly as a result of the first wave of massive immigration from the Islamic countries, equality of educational opportunity acquired first priority status on the list of educational issues. Following independence, the absorption of immigrants became the primary concern of the state. These immigrants' ideological commitment to Zionism could no longer be taken for granted.

Many came because they had been persecuted in the Arab countries after Israel gained its independence. Even the newer immigrants from Europe, tired and disillusioned after the Nazi Holocaust, brought a predominantly present-orientation to their new homeland. In terms of the basic difference in values—communal-idealistic versus—familistic-traditional—the ineffectiveness of the kibbutz based residential schools in absorbing these postwar children who arrived with their families became obvious.

In the light of the change in the return of immigration, residential education was formally divorced from the now increasingly particularistic ideological climate of the kibbutz and became an institutionalized branch of the national educational system, with Youth Aliyah as an ongoing partner. Nevertheless, a dualism became apparent in view of the continued adherence of the residential educational system to the perpetuation of agriculture as an ideal. Others came to see these values as less necessary in the upbringing of the young generation, who were no longer expected to emulate the qualities of the glorified culture hero, the "chalutz" or pioneer. Nevertheless, the agricultural ethos was still considered to have intrinsic educational value.

This makes sense within the context of modern Jewish history. Back in 1882, Leo Pinsker stressed the "inverted Pyramid" of occupations observable in European Jewish communities; i.e., the heavy emphasis on bookishness, the high concentration in the professions and commerce, and the lack of involvement in physical labor. Though rooted in Jewish heritage, the Zionists, as members of a national movement, strove to disassociate themselves from the anomalies of Diaspora existence. To remedy this "unhealthy" socio-economic structure, the pioneers dedicated themselves to physical labor, especially agriculture. This line of thinking resulted, during the pre-statehood period, in an overall anti-intellectual atmosphere among the settlers. They were motivated by a mixture of neo-physiocratic belief in the value of the land and an emotional insistence on striking roots in a new-old land.

As earlier stated, this romanticized view of an agrarian culture which emerged in the newly created State had only slight resemblance to the reality of a rapidly changing, industrialized, technologically oriented urban society. Within this framework, specialized education gained ascendancy and replaced the previously held ideal of a generalist or universal education (Wolins, 1971).

Within the context of an ethnically heterogeneous society absorbing massive immigration from East and West, the provision of equal educational opportunity becomes a paramount, but clearly problematic, social issue. The residential alternative was one of the major educational means for achieving this goal that the educational system tried. Prevailing philosophies of immigrant absorption rooted in the melting pot model encouraged the adoption of a differential pace of acculturation for the various generations within the immigrant family (Frankenstein, 1951). Thus the removal of talented youngsters was encouraged on the basis of the assumption that they could be socialized to the norms of their new homeland more effectively in residential schools than in their original family settings (Frankenstein, 1961; Rottenschtreich, 1951).

Lack of concern for the immigrant family as a unit proved to be detrimental, however, both for the immigrants and for the absorbing society. Intergenerational tension, alienation, and uprootedness of both the young and the old were byproducts of this policy. This was reflected in intense interethnic tension that gradually became politicized and exploded two and a half decades later during the mid and late 1970s in a variety of new political alignments.

The nature of residential education also changed in that the institution was no longer called upon to fulfill an *in loco parentis* role because most of their parents had also immigrated. Nevertheless many institutions continued to see socialization and character formation as their primary educational objective, although most programs had added a vocational education component as well. The latter was considered to be of minor, or, at best, secondary importance by the staffs (Smilansky, Kashti, & Arieli, 1982). The great majority of students in residential care from the fifties onwards were of Sephar-origin, however, and both the parents' and the students' main interest lay in the career-oriented component of these programs, which they viewed as their chance for integration and upward mobility in the rapidly changing Israeli society. This goal ambiguity undermined considerably the parental mandate which the institutions enjoyed.

Thus, the traditional socialization or character formation goal of the institution became increasingly problematic. The melting pot model of absorption has been gradually replaced by a pluralistic approach recognizing the need to examine and accommodate to, if not reinforce, systematically the various newcomers' cultures of origin. Becoming familiar with their family support systems, decision making processes, parenting styles and intergenerational relations were all seen as crucial in helping new immigrants settle in (Eilam, 1980;

Eisikovits and Adam, 1981). Only by taking these elements and associated parental expectations for their children's educational outcomes into consideration in designing the residential environment could the institution be developed as a socially adaptive answer to its client population needs.

A discrepancy between the traditional "normalcy" ideology of institutional education in Israel and the emerging needs of student populations became apparent. A great many residential settings did not diversify their programs in accordance with changing student exigencies, nor did they, in fact, attract sufficiently high quality manpower to be able to perform such a complex task. Although dealing with a multi-problem population, the youth counselors ("madrichim") were no longer the high-prestige, broadly-educated pioneers of the pre-statehood days (Wolins, 1971), when they served as role models socializing their charges to an ideology and a life style. The career of youth counselor had gradually dwindled into a negative or, at best, transient status which, in turn, contributed to the further downward spiraling of the quality of education offered.

Further, the once-heterogenous student body that included day students from surrounding communities who were attracted to the institutions by the high reputation of their programs has been undergoing a process of homogenization. Lack of ongoing communication with the outside community contributed to the further isolation of the institution and a decline in its dynamism and ability to serve as an equalizer of educational opportunity.

Indeed, Smilansky, Kashti, and Arieli (1982, pp. 132-3) note that a considerable number of institutions surveyed in their recent study run at high vacancy levels caused by low enrollments and high dropout rates. They claim that in the past two decades a considerable number of good community schools offering a variety of vocational training programs have been established in many development towns traditionally inhabited by a high concentration of new immigrant populations. This means that placing youth in residential schools for their education and particularly for technical training is no longer the only alternative. They also point to a basic incompatibility between potential candidates in real need of placement and the willingness of institutions to accommodate them, since these settings are often reluctant to admit predelinquent youths for fear of further compromising their waning status as "normative educational options" with academic aspirations. Furthermore, they lack staff properly qualified to deal with the special needs of these students.

CONCLUSION

It is clear that residential education in Israel has reached a critical juncture. In the pre-statehood days the institution served as a cultural "maximizer" (Henry, 1965) for its charges due to the congruence between its particularistic goals and the larger universal values of the pioneering society. Following statehood, residential education underwent a crisis as its traditional normative educational/socialization ideology was challenged by the rapidly changing demographic picture in the larger, ethnically heterogeneous society, for which the formation of an "ideal type" or "modal character" Israeli became decreasingly adaptive.

The institution is caught between nostalgia for its glorious past and the need for radical change in some of its basic approaches as a precondition for its survival. By preferring the perpetuation of traditional goals and organizational structures to the introduction of substantive changes in the interest of their current clientele, many of these institutions have become cultural "minimizers," unable to perform adequately the task for which they have been given a social mandate: to equip new, "disadvantaged" immigrant youth with better coping skills for functioning in the larger society. This brings us back to our initial premise where, in contradiction with Yehudi Cohen's skeptical view about man's ability to influence deliberately the "emergency or loss" of cultural institutions, we maintain that, by controlling their character, one is actually passing a verdict on an institution's very existence. The evolution of the Israeli residential school is a case in point.

The study of one social institution, Cohen has claimed, yields valuable insights into macro-social processes. What can we learn about Israeli society from the foregoing longitudinal analysis of the functions of residential education? Its present impasse reflects the dilemmas of the larger society regarding the equitable handling of the plethora of problems stemming from ethnic and cultural differences. Lacking the clarity of vision that characterized its earlier days, the residential school of the present is called upon to operationalize a yet uncrystallized social philosophy.

REFERENCES

Bowlby, J. (1952). Maternal care and mental health. (2nd Ed.). Geneva: World Health Organization.

Bronfenbrenner, U. (1970). Two worlds of childhood: U.S. and U.S.S.R. New York: Russell Sage Foundation.

Cohen, Y. A. (1975). The state system, schooling and cognitive and motivational patterns. In N. K. Shimahara & A. Scrupski (Eds.), *Social forces and schooling: An anthropological and sociological perspective*. New York: David McKay Company, Inc.

Eilam, Y. (1980). *The Georgians in Israel: Anthropological perspectives*. Jerusalem: Hebrew University (in Hebrew).

Eisenstadt, S. N. (1967). *Israeli society*. London: Weidenfeld and Nicolson.

Eisikovits, R., & Adam, V. (1981). The social integration of new immigrant children from the Caucasus in Israeli schools. *Studies in Education, 31* (in Hebrew).

Frankenstein, K. (1951). To the problem of ethnic differences. *Megamot, 2*, 261-276 (in Hebrew).

Frankenstein, K. (1961). The school without parents. *Megamot, 12*, 3-23 (in Hebrew).

Henry, J. (1965). *Culture against man*. New York: Vintage Books.

Kashti, Y. (1979). *The socializing community: Disadvantaged adolescents in Israeli youth villages*. Tel-Aviv University: The School of Education.

Kashti, Y., Arieli, M., & Wozner, Y. (1981). The Israeli residential setting: Tradition, social context, organization. In Report of the Israeli-American Seminar on Out-of-School Education, *Residential education in Israel*. Jerusalem: The Ministry of Education and Culture.

King, E. J. (1974). *Other schools and ours*. (4th Ed.). London: Holt, Rinehart and Winston.

Kleinberger, A. F. (1969). *Society, school and progress in Israel*. New York: Pergamon Press.

Pinsker, L. (1882). *Auto-Emancipation*. Berlin: Privately published (mimeo).

Rottenschtreich, N. (1951). Absolute measures. *Megamot, 2*, 327-338 (in Hebrew).

Smilansky, M., Kashti, Y., & Arieli, M. (1982). *The residential education alternative*. Haifa: Ach Publishing House.

Wallace, A. F. C. (1961). Schools in revolutionary and conservative societies. In F. C. Gruber (Ed.), *Anthropology and education*. Philadelphia: University of Pennsylvania Press.

Weeks, A. L. (1974). Boarding schools in the U.S.S.R. In M. Wolins (Ed.), *Successful group care: Explorations in the powerful environment*. Chicago: Aldine.

Wolins, M. (Ed.). (1974). *Successful group care: Explorations in the powerful environment*. Chicago: Aldine.

Wolins, M. (1971). Youth Aliyah: Cause and function. In M. Wolins and M. Gottesman (Eds.), *Group care: An Israeli approach* (pp. 3-26). New York: Gordon & Breach.

Wolins, M., & Gottesman, M. (Eds.). (1971). *Group care: An Israeli approach*. New York: Gordon & Breach.

II.

Programmatic Expressions

Institutional Placement:
An Interim Stage or an End in Itself?:
The Role of Parents
in the Continuum of Care

Zmira Laufer

ABSTRACT. Research has supported the general professional consensus that, to be most effective, an institutional placement program must maintain the cooperation and involvement of a child's parents. Nonetheless, and despite policy mandates in this direction, one of the most neglected aspects in the process of child care in Israel is the linkage between the family and the institution. To illuminate this need and problem, the following includes a short summary of theory and research on the impact of parent-institution relationships on the child's development; a description of the current situation in Israel in this regard, including the degree of cooperation between social workers in the community and the institution and their relationships with the child and his family; a discussion of the conflicts inherent in maintaining a child placement organization with the goal of returning children to their homes as quickly as feasible; and discussion and recommendation of means of improving cooperation and communication among those involved in the placement process and, thus, achieving more of the officially stated aims of child placement.

Current research suggests that an effective program for the placement of a child outside his or her parents' home must rely on the parents' involvement and cooperation. While child welfare workers in Israel tend to agree, in actual practice involvement of and cooperation between the parents and the institution suffers from considerable neglect. The present paper focuses on this issue.

Theory and research on the development of children's institutions and the outcomes of their treatment programs use two common clas-

Zmira Laufer, School of Social Work, University of Haifa, Mount Carmel, Haifa 31 999, Israel.

33

sifications, one dividing institutions according to the age of the population they serve (e.g., adolescent institutions), and the other dividing the institutions according to the stated reason for the original placement (e.g., mental retardation, delinquency, etc.). A widely accepted classification of the latter type is that devised by Kadushin (1974, pp. 617-618), covering five types of institutions according to children's specific needs at a certain age:

— institutions for normal but dependent and neglected children;
— institutions for physically handicapped children (blindness, etc.);
— institutions for mentally retarded or mentally defective children;
— institutions for the confinement and rehabilitation of juvenile delinquents;
— institutions for emotionally disturbed children.

Any classification related to the Israeli situation has to take into account two important parameters, namely length of stay and legal status of the child, from which four categories may be defined: children placed for a definitive period or as an intermediate stage in treatment following the parents' consent; children placed for a prolonged period, or permanently (severe retardation, etc.); children placed against the parents' will following a court order for brief or prolonged definite periods of time; and children whose parents have been permanently deprived of their custody rights and who are waiting for adoption or another alternative.

In the first two groups, the children are essentially under the parents' guardianship since the placement is implemented with their consent. In the second group the law intervenes due to the need to protect the child's interest, and as a result the parents' rights are taken away, either for a short period or permanently.

Most of the children of different ages who have been placed in Israeli institutions belong to the first legal category and are under the care of three governmental bodies: the Youth Immigration Authority, which has placed the largest number of children older than primary school age; the Child and Youth Service in the Ministry of Welfare, which has placed the largest number of pre-school and primary-school children; and the Ministry of Education, which has been responsible for the development of children's boarding schools.

It seems important to focus on pre- and primary school children firstly because of their extreme vulnerability, in the light of researchers' emphasis on the finding that the younger the child is, the more vital the family framework, and secondly because of the fact that children of this age are not able to initiate ties with their parents through their own efforts and depend for this on the initiative of the various professionals (Cohen, 1972; Weiner, 1979, Ch. 7). Nevertheless, some of the issues to be discussed bear significance for children from other age groups in similar family situations.

After reviewing theory and research in the area of parent-child relationship in the context of placement, the basic stages in placement of children outside their homes in Israel, the treatment aspects involved, and the method used to treat the child and his family during the child's stay in the institution will be discussed. Implications of existing interaction between the various participants in the placement program, and the relevant recommendations for the future will be drawn.

THE PARENT-CHILD RELATIONSHIP AND THE INSTITUTIONAL SYSTEM

The issue of continuing ties between the child and his parents during the child's stay in a setting outside the home is of constant concern to those occupied with the child's welfare. While in the past the generally preferred approach was to "save children from their parents" in the belief that physical separation would sever the emotional and psychological ties between them, reality has demonstrated the error of this assumption; it is impossible to eliminate the ties between a child and his family even when they are most disorganized or detrimental (Simmons et al., 1973).

Littner (1975) lists four primary reasons that explain why a child's ties with his biological parents remain important even when the child is placed with foster parents or in institutions. The child feels the absence of his parents and misses them even if their relations are disturbed and difficult because he is still dependent upon them for providing him with a source of security. Secondly, a child removed from his home has no understanding of the reasons why he has been made to leave his parents and he imagines a series of irrational explanations such as, for example, that because he has been a bad boy he has been taken out of the home. Thirdly, the child identified with his parents in such a way that any criticism directed towards them, justified or not, is viewed by the child as an attack on himself. A fourth reason is that while separated from parents, the child may develop an incorrect image of them, whether positive or negative, and of himself or herself as a consequence.

In the present context we should add an additional reason for maintaining ties between parents and children that involves the agreement drawn up with the parents whereby they are to assume certain parental roles from time to time (e.g., decisions on medical treatment, receiving the child for vacations, etc.). Further, parental ties are known to be necessary for the child's development and achievements in the new setting, for working on the possibility and timing of the child's return to the home, and the methods by which the institutions can contribute to the improvement of parental functioning.

Matsusima (1965) refers to the implications of parent-child ties, stating that "the paramount advantage of contact with parents is the continuous reality of parental proximity of the child." In Matsusima's opinion, preventing parent-child ties and encounters can only harm the child's capacity to benefit from the institutional care.

Moss (1969) focuses on the separation between parents and children and states that a lack of attention to parent-child ties harms both the child's capacity for adaptation to the institution and his ability to benefit from the opportunities available because of the trauma of separation upon entrance and the repeated need for separation at each visit coupled with ignorance of the need to shape a new parent-child relationship. Children are in constant need of proof of their parents' love and of their place in the family. The establishment of a modified relationship that is clear to the child helps him to cope with this need and permits the development of positive ties with others. The possibility of transforming the separation process into a positive event is discussed by Wilkes (1980), who states that a proper attitude can transform this process into a unifying act that can contribute to the child's self-esteem.

A comparative study carried out by Simmons et al. (1973) on three groups of children placed in institutions revealed that children whose parents visited the institution regularly and participated in institutional life and activities reached higher academic achievements, a more strongly developed self-concept, stronger ties to their biological families, and a better capacity to establish friendships. Secondly, they found that these parents exhibited more functional attitudes towards their children and enhanced general parental performance.

The effects of regular parent-child contact on the timing of children's return home has been investigated by Fanshel (1975) in a five-year study covering 624 children placed in institutions. His findings indicate that the frequency of visits is closely associated with the child's probability of returning home in a short time.

The view of the institution as a locus for improved parental functioning and developing parental skills, seem to hold great promise. Such a view requires that institutional admissions policies be set so that only children whose parents can easily visit the institution can qualify for admission. As early as 1965, Matsusima (1965) describes the implementation of such a policy in a residential facility where admission was limited to the immediate county population. Likewise, it should be stated by policy that treating the child's family is also the task of the institution.

In recent years, a number of varied experiments where parents were involved in the institutional treatment process have been published, reporting considerable success both in terms of improved parenthood and long-term effects (e.g., Simmons et al., 1973; Williams, 1972; Magnus, 1974; Kamerman and Kahn, 1981; Littauer, 1980; Wood, 1981).

In sum, there is much support for the idea that the parental role is a crucial one in the development of young people in placement. What follows is a description of actual practice in Israel to be examined from this perspective.

STAGES IN REMOVING CHILDREN FROM THEIR HOMES

While the family in Israel is highly valued, the percentage of children living away from home in Israel is extremely high compared to that in other developed countries. Approximately 6% of all children under the age of eighteen are in boarding schools. The manifest purpose of many of these placements is to separate the children from the negative influence of their families, which are unable to function adequately and to fulfill the children's needs, especially in the area of education (Honig and Shamai, 1978).

In recent years two salient changes can be seen in the approach to institutional placement of children (0-14 years) following their parents' neglect and inability to function (Laufer, 1980).

First, children's emotional needs have achieved equal status with their educational needs; when decisions are made with regard to removal from the home, the two need systems are both taken into consideration. Secondly, while the institution continues to be accepted in Israel as the best response to the educational needs of children who can no longer continue to be raised in their parent's home, there is no longer the same level of expectation that the institution will fulfill emotional needs as well.

It seems that one of the important sources for these shifts lies in the changes that occurred in the profile of professionals working in the area of child welfare. In the past, child welfare workers came largely from education backgrounds, both at the policy-making and at the direct care work levels. Today, these two levels are populated by personnel with social work, psychology and counseling backgrounds. They have in common a professional ideology emphasizing the need for an emotional foundation prior to educational achievement. Since the residential program is no longer seen as providing an efficient way to meet this need, greater attention is being given to the role of the child's home and family.

A decision to place outside the home is usually made at the primary stage by the social worker who is in direct contact with the family, his/her direct superior in the local agency (the supervisor or director), and by a regional consultant from the Child and Youth Service Department in the Ministry of Welfare.[1] For certain groups such as pre-school children, an additional Child and Youth Service committee reviews the need to remove the child from his home due to the special significance of the separation from their parents of children at this age (Laufer, 1980).

Recent experience suggests that the participants in the decision to remove a child from the home usually expect this treatment alternative to fulfill the following of the entire range of parental functions: preserve the child's physical security; provide him with housing, nourishment, education, and enrichment; care for him during physical illness; and follow up on and help the child with any emotional difficulties. Parents, on the other hand, are expected to provide continuity in the child's sense of belonging, to take responsibility in case of major medical intervention (i.e., surgery), to provide a home as an alternative to the institution during vacations or in transitional stages from one institution to another, and to participate in

---

[1]A somewhat different but analogous process occurs in assigning children to institutions under the auspices of the Ministry of Education.

maintenance costs according to their capacity, with the under-standing that the Ministry of Welfare will pay the difference. Thus, the various persons involved in the treatment plan aim to develop a situation of shared and complementary parenthood for the child in-volving the biological parents, the residential care workers, and the local social service agency.

The period of time allotted for the residential alternative is for-mally defined as an "interim stage" during which the child will re-main in the institution until a change occurs in the family's function-ing to enable it to re-accept the child. In reality, however, in light of their practice experience, the social workers tend to see this ar-rangement as lasting at least until the child reaches adulthood. The gap between the manifest, formal bureaucratic definition of the situation and latent expectations will be discussed later.

It must be recalled that the structure of most of Israel's institu-tions also reinforces the "interim stage" approach in child place-ment. Most are designed for a specific age group or a specific ed-ucational level, so that as the child reaches a certain age and a new educational level, he must be transferred to an institution with an educational program that will respond to his needs.

What are the implications of the "interim stage" factor in the current placement scene in Israel? Once the decision to place the child outside his home has been made by the human service profes-sionals with the parents' consent, a parent is required to sign two forms: a parental consent form and a contract with the Ministry tak-ing responsibility for placing the child. The tone of the contract reflects the anticipated treatment process once the child is outside the home, and hence deserves some attention.

A central aspect of this contract is the financial arrangement be-tween the Ministry of Welfare and the parents (six paragraphs out of a total of twenty). A second major section deals with the legal aspects of the actual signing and the fulfillment or non-fulfillment of the conditions of the contract (six paragraphs). The obligations of the Ministry of Welfare are defined in only two paragraphs, one stating the services to be provided by the Ministry to the child, and the second stating the Ministry's duty to notify the parents upon ter-mination of the treatment, or upon the decision to transfer the child to another institution. Six other paragraphs refer to cooperation re-quired from the parents; the parents must notify the Ministry of any change in their address or family situation, promise to obey institu-tional rules, accept the child for vacations during fixed periods determined by the institution, remove the child in case he is found unsuitable to the institution, accept responsibility in case of special medical treatment or surgical intervention, and grant power-of-attorney to the Ministry of Welfare to transfer the child from place to place following prior notice.

The name of the institution where the child will be placed is not included, nor is there any specification of the amount of time within which the Ministry promises to propose placement. The Ministry is under no obligation to report to the parents on its activities with regard to implementation of the terms of the contract; that is, the Ministry does not have to report on positive or negative developments throughout the institutional placement. The sole obligation to notify the parents occurs when the child is transferred from one institution to another, and even then there is no stipulation as to the amount of time the parents are given for filing reservations or complaints.

Another salient point is that at the time the contract is signed, the parents do not actually know what action is expected of them in connection with the institution; they must maintain "existing arrangements," which remain undefined, or receive the child at home during vacations dictated by the institution—again an undefined demand. Thus, parents make commitments that they are not sure they will be able to fulfill. It should be noted that the social worker does not know whether the parents will be able to live up to future demands or duties either, since he or she cannot know what these will consist of at a time when the institution where the child will be placed has not yet been determined.

The duration of the contract is one year, but it is renewed automatically for an additional year. This means that when the contract is renewed there is no need for both sides to meet and discuss the developments that have arisen during the year in addition to possible changes in conditions for the following year.

In summary, the contract that formalizes ties and cooperation between the parents and the authorities responsible for the child's care is unclear, and it emphasizes the parents' obligations towards the Ministry of Welfare and the institution towards the parents. In addition, it is evident that the contract emphasizes the temporariness of the arrangement while simultaneously leaving the time period for care undefined; that is, it may be said that the message it carries is that placement outside the home is a "chronic transitional stage."

Following the completion of the forms, which include the social worker's report, usually a psychologist's report on the results of an

intelligence test, and medical certificates, the decision on the particular institution where the child will be placed is made by an
authorized committee or consultant. Two important factors in Israeli
reality must be mentioned here: first, in most cases the children are
not placed in their home communities; secondly, in most cases,
there is no combined treatment provided for the parents and the
child following placement, and parental treatment, if any, occurs
under the auspices of the community service.

Orientation procedures differ from one institution to another, and
usually a visit is made to the institution by the child accompanied by
a parent and a social worker from the community agency. In cases
where the parents are uncooperative or handicapped in some way,
the child is accompanied by the social worker alone. The nature of
this visit also differs according to the institution, but in most cases
an emphasis is placed on getting to know the physical layout of the
place. At this preliminary orientation stage, the institutions usually
have the right to accept or reject the placement candidate. It is note-
worthy that the workers responsible for the child's treatment in the
past and in the future are not required to set a schedule for continued
parent-child contact. Another point is that not all relevant information about parents may be provided to the institution by the community worker due to apprehension that such information may harm
the child's chance to be accepted by the institution.

THE CHILD, HIS PARENTS, THE INSTITUTION,
AND COMMUNITY WELFARE SERVICES
DURING PLACEMENT

Consensus exists among professonals involved in child placement
in Israeli institutions that stable parent-child ties influence positively
the child's development in the institution. Furthermore, both community and institutional workers give lip-service to their shared
obligation to actively take part in developing these ties. In the light
of the above it is important to examine existing means for maintaining parent-child ties and communication channels between professionals in the community and the residential setting.

Means for Continuous Parent-Child Ties During Residential Care

In most of the institutions under the supervision of the Child and
Youth Service of the Ministry of Welfare, three communication
methods are recommended but not required: home visits during

vacations and holidays, parents' visits to the institution, and letters and telephone calls.

Home Visits. Each institution maintains its own policy on home visits, depending on the treatment approach adopted by the institution. Some are strict about the frequency of visits, some decide on arrangements based on the individual needs of the child and his family, and some permit visits based on technical considerations such as staff vacations. Prior to the visit, some institutions contact the community service to request follow-up and a report on the visit. Some send staff members to visit the child and his parents at home; others do not take an interest in the quality of the visit.

Sometimes children cannot be sent home for reasons such as the parents' hospitalization, instability, etc., and the institutions adopt several alternative approaches in dealing with such situations. Some see it as their duty to locate an alternative arrangement for the child, and they may find staff members' families, for example, who are prepared to host children during these times; others allow the children to remain at the institution with a reduced staff or find a foster family for the vacation. There are some institutions where this is perceived as the task of the community service, and in such cases the local agency is expected to find a suitable family for the child to stay with.

Attitudes toward home visits also vary. In some institutions, children are encouraged to go home for visits, and special attention is paid to the children's external appearance before the visit, they are equipped with small gifts for the parents, pocket money, provisions for the road, and transportation services. Furthermore, an investment is made in initiating contact with the local welfare agency on this issue. Other institutions see the home visit as a "necessary evil," stating that the child returns from home in emotional crisis with wild behavior. Even physically, he may not return in the same condition as when he was sent home; he often returns with lice or some other symptom of physical neglect, and he receives many presents from his parents which later arouse envy among the other children. In short, following each home visit, they feel treatment must be started anew. Thus, although home visits are usually seen as a viable means for maintaining continuity in parent-child ties during institutionalization, some residential settings do not take advantage of them and perceive them as hampering the results of the previous institutional care.

Sometimes the child receives a double message from the institution on this issue. The source of such situations lies in differences in the professional level, knowledge, and skills of the staff members. While staff members like the institutional director, the social worker, and the educational advisor normally understand the significance of the home visit and actively encourage it, those responsible for direct care—the child care workers, the housemothers, teachers—are unaware of the potential for treatment arising from such encounters and fail to make full use of them as therapeutic situations.

Parental Visits to the Institution. A wide range of programs for parental visits to the institution may be found, varying according to the institutional perception of its role in the process of shared parenthood. Frequently a specific visiting day is set for all parents, when the institution prepared to receive them by organizing a special program of entertainment, provides an opportunity for them to meet staff members, and allows for the parents to spend time with their children and "wander around the grounds." Another method of organizing group visits is to invite the parents to special events held at the institution—celebrations, group bar mitzvahs, etc.

There are some institutions that use the group visit primarily in order to "put on a show" of "quality care" to impress the parents, while others emphasize the role the parents play in the treatment process by granting them an opportunity for questions and conversation with the various staff members and residents. The predetermination of a common parents' visiting day is thrifty in terms of the manpower investment required by the institution, but it has little effectiveness in terms of communication between parents, children, and the institution.

Individually arranged visits for parents seem to be more effective towards enhanced communication and continuity in parents' involvement with their child's institutional experience. Some institutions are opting for visits on a "whenever the parent decides to come" basis. While these seem to be less efficient, they also provide a wide range of possibilities for potential involvement.

The Child and Youth Service is opting for a policy of encouraging parental visiting, reaching out to inform and convince parents of its importance. Financial resources have been budgeted to provide transportation to the institution for parents who do not have the means to pay. It is important, however, to recall that the implementation of this policy remains optional both for parents and the institution, resulting in a wide variety of levels of parental involvement.

This is problematic if one accepts that parental involvement is a promising indicator of the future possibilities of returning the child home or, alternatively, withdrawing parental rights completely.

Letters and Telephone Calls. In spite of their potential to maintain communication, these channels are not utilized optimally. This is due by and large to parents' not having a phone and being unable or unwilling to write. On the other hand, workers in the community can and should initiate such communication, and when they do it exists. Given the importance of collaboration between community and institutional professionals this and other areas will be addressed next.

Communication Between Community Service and the Residential Facility. Most of Israel's institutions today employ social workers who maintain contact with the referring welfare agency from the community and treating the child's parents is one of their central tasks. This section focuses on the relationship between the community social worker and those associated with the residential agency.

The recommendations laid down by the Ministry of Welfare state that this contact should be achieved through periodic mutual reports on the child's development and progress in the institution. Such collaboration is seen as essential due to their different foci of family functioning. On the basis of this joint assessment the need for continuing institutionalization is expected to be reviewed periodically.

Contact between the two is also necessary due to the division of parental roles between the institution and the parents, as described above. Thus, for example, the institutional social worker usually expects his colleague in the community to make sure the parents will accept the child for vacations, to encourage them to come to the visiting days at the institution, to take care of various formal papers, etc. The community social worker expects his institutional colleagues to encourage the child to write, to help find an alternative arrangement to the parents' home should a crisis arise that might prevent the child from coming home for vacation, etc. That is, both expect complementary actions regarding the fulfillment of the child's needs.

In practice, the workers often see themselves as working on opposite sides of the track. For the community social worker and the parent, the child's placement outside the home signals a sense of failure arising from exhausting all alternative means. For the worker, the institutional placement of the child may be seen more as an end in itself in removing a "thorn in the side" of the agency, rather than as a "transitional stage" in treatment. This is reinforced by the fact that the continuing treatment program for parents is not formally required and, that follow-up with families whose children have been placed is not taken into account in determining the social worker's caseload.

As for contact with the institution, the worker frequently feels completely uninformed about developments there and, although he or she must make reports to the institution and take care of various technical matters regarding the placement, the institution is not pressured to make its reports to the community worker. The resulting situation often gives the social worker the feeling of being a "messenger boy." Another frequent claim is that the community social worker is "stuck" with all the severe cases and the accompanying frustration of working with problematic parents, yet does not receive the same credit granted to the institutional staff members who gain success and satisfaction from working with children who reach demonstrable achievements. Thus, the community social worker often feels trapped between the alternative of taking responsibility for permanent separation of the child from his home by putting him up for irreversible placement, and that of continuing to work with a family in relation to which the worker feels "burned out," and in concert with an institution that produces a feeling of alienation.

In contrast, the institutional social worker begins his acquaintance with the child's parents through the community social worker's report, which usually outlines extensively the parents' weaknesses and their negative influence on the child's development while giving little or no space to their strengths. Nor is there a discussion of the positive aspects of the past parent-child relationship, or plans to continue this relationship or modify it. This report, along with the child himself, who often presents a whole series of difficulties, creates conscious or unconscious *a priori* hostility toward the parents and also provokes the idea that the child must be "saved" from them. These feelings contradict the institutional social worker's knowledge of the importance of the parent-child ties and their implications for the positive use of the child's stay in the institution. It is thus reasonable to assume that, at the beginning of the road, the social worker already has a built-in conflict concerning the parents.

During the child's stay in the institution, the worker must deal with a range of demands imposed by the parents and the community service, often with resulting "interference" in the treatment program implemented within the institution. A complaint frequently voiced by social workers is the feeling that community services do not cooperate adequately. The institutional workers are meanwhile essentially unaware of the financial and treatment limitations binding the community workers, and they are not sufficiently familiar with the child's home. In this regard, it must be recalled that the communication patterns recommended by the Child and Youth Service for smooth cooperation between the two are just that—a recommendation. An additional source of conflict arising among institutional social workers and other staff members is that an improvement in the child's or the parents' functioning, and the initiation of meaningful ties between them may mean the child's leaving the institution and breaking established relationships. This may present a problem for the worker as well as the child in terms of termination of treatment and other issues.

An additional obstacle for the institutional social worker in collaborating with his community service colleague lies in the former's historical lack of appreciation for the level of professional work done in the community. Working on the behalf of his client—in this case, the child, with whom he identifies—the institutional worker finds it difficult to accept the perceived lack of greater professional competence and accordingly develops a feeling of disdain for his local colleague. This situation is perpetuated by the continuing low level of professional performance in local public welfare agencies.

In order to round the picture of the institutional social worker's attitude towards the child's parents, it must be added that most institutions view their social workers as primarily in charge of the children's emotional adjustment to institutional life rather than maintaining ties with factors outside the institutions. Accordingly the number of slots allotted for social workers is low. The Ministry of Welfare's regulation establishes a social work position for every one hundred children in institutions for "regular" populations or a worker for every thirty or forty children in pre-school or other specialized institutions. In spite of this, maintaining contact with the children's families falls within the responsibility of the social worker.

DISCUSSION AND RECOMMENDATIONS

In analyzing the processes involved in placing a child in an institution in Israel, and in maintaining parental ties under such circumstances, we have seen that participation by the child, the parents, and the various professionals at the institution and in the community welfare service is involved. Any such collaborative effort requires careful attention to the development of efficient communication methods that will permit coping with changes over time, and to the clarification of role definitions that will make explicit the various tasks of each participant in relation to the others. In the placement process as it currently exists in Israel, however, all of the crucial roles seem to be unclear.

Further, it has been demonstrated that level of output increases when a worker is provided with a clear definition and a quantitative measure of what is expected of him, and that output declines when such a definition is lacking (Steers and Porter, 1979; Locke et al., 1981). Thus, tasks that are not quantitatively defined in the treatment program will not be optimally accomplished. In the present context, for example, the lack of specified number of required home visits and required parental visits to the institution, or a required frequency of communication among the various staff members involved with the young person and the family inevitably leads to a low level of performance in each of these tasks. In addition, in light of the complementary nature of the tasks performed by each participant, the lack of preset rules leads to the development of expectations based on each participant's individual perceptions, expectations that are neither agreed upon nor frequently realizable; the result is frustration and claimed lack of cooperation on all sides.

The urgent need to adopt a policy of clear, mandatory goal-setting and appropriate means of control is evidenced by the fact that, despite the recommendations and guidelines set forth by the Child and Youth Service for the purpose of maintaining the ties among the institution, the parents, and the community service, their implementation is spotty (Ministry of Labor, 1977). Moreover, scholars dealing with complex organizations in a dynamic environment emphasize that utmost attention must be devoted to the development of communication channels between the organization and the environment in order for the organization's plans to be flexible and able to adapt to change (Hall, 1972). Yet, there is no continuous, multidirectional reporting going on among the community service, the parents, and the institution. Even if the Child and Youth Services' recommendations are fully implemented through periodic reports, they will not fully respond to the need to obtain information in such a complex and changing environment.

The lack of adequate communication may also be viewed in light of the well-known effects of feedback on performance. In the new approaches to motivation, feedback is the indispensable *a priori* condition for improving performance or raising the level of output (Locke, 1981; Erez, 1977). Since the tasks are complementary, the feedback requirement applies to all the participants in these tasks.

Another central problem that interferes with the effectiveness of the treatment program is the difficulty the participants face in determining a time frame for its completion. In most cases, all participants agree that the shared parenthood program is an intermediate stage and that, following the achievement of the goal of improving parental functioning, the child should be returned home and the placement program terminated. In actual practice, however, institutions have been unsuccessful in developing any criteria for determining the length of stay; in most cases, children and their parents are left in "limbo" and the institutionalization becomes more an end in itself than a means. This tendency is further reinforced by the option left to institutions to renew the placement contract automatically. The child is placed "intermediately," but actually indefinitely.

To resolve the problem of a "chronic intermediate stage," it appears that there is a need to change the existing approaches to institutional treatment in Israel in fundamental ways. First, change is needed in the perception of the placement process and institutional treatment as the focus of the program, whereas only secondary importance is attached to working with the parents; both processes should be given the same level of consideration and importance. In this connection, urgent attention should be given to the development of programs to improve the parenting skills of families whose children have been placed in institutions. The period of institutionalization will be "intermediate" only if material and therapeutic resources are invested in the parents so that they are helped to improve their functioning.

Only the community service operates in this area today. In light of the tendency for family caseworkers to reach the institutional placement stage when they have burned out on a particular case, perhaps a different worker should be assigned to the family once the child has been placed outside the home. Presently, the dominant approach is that turnover of caseworkers should be avoided for individual cases, and that the more extensive the worker's contact with the family, the better. While it is indeed true that rapid turnover may be harmful, turnover that follows the termination of one stage of treatment and the beginning of another, as in the case of a child placed outside the home, may have positive effects: the worker who has experienced burnout and has exhausted his treatment potential with a particular family can be replaced by a new worker who is fresh to the case and not burdened by less than successful prior experiences.

From the many attempts that have been made in various countries to enhance parental effectiveness, as described in the introductory section above, it is evident that such parent education programs are often quite successful when their locus is in the institution itself. In Israel, the parents' geographically limited access to the institution presents an obstacle in the development of such programs. However, the notion that the locus of parental treatment should be the institution should lead to a policy change whereby the institutions are serving families from the surrounding area rather than a larger regional or national clientele. As a transitional stage toward this policy, workers should currently ensure the placement of children in institutions near their home communities.

Another change that should be made is in the structure of institutions in Israel. As described above, many of the institutions are specialized in a certain age group. Under such conditions, children are repeatedly referred from one institution to another as they grow up. Therefore, group care facilities should be expected to serve a wider age range of children and adolescents together. An additional step that should be taken is to require periodic assessment, based on clear, pre-existing criteria, for termination or continuation of placement to avoid unnecessary long-term institutionalization.

In summary, it may be said that the present paper constitutes an attempt to map the factors responsible for the fact that, in many cases, child placement in Israel has, despite official declarations to the contrary, become a "chronic intermediate stage" in which the role of the parents in healthy child development tends to be ignored. The paper suggests that this does not reflect a lack of understanding of the importance of the parental role and the family, but rather the difficulty in applying this knowledge in practice in the context of the child welfare system as it is currently organized. Therefore, it seems that what is needed now is the establishment of a systematic effort to assess approaches to child placement in order to ensure the application of the idea that removing the child from the home is only the first step in a treatment prescription and rarely, if ever, an end in itself.

REFERENCES

Adoption of Children Law 5741-1981. In *Sefer Ha Chukkim,* No. 1928, 24th Iyar, 5741, pp. 293 (in Hebrew).

Cohen, M. (1972). A survey of institutional infants in need of parents. *SAAD, 6,* 91-102 (in Hebrew).

Erez, M. (1977). A necessary condition for the goal-setting performance relationship. *Journal of Applied Psychology, 64,* 349-371.

Fanshel, D. (1975). Parental visiting of children in foster care: Key to discharge? *Social Service Review, 49,* 493-514.

Hall, R. H. (1972). *Organizations—structure and process.* Englewood Cliffs, New Jersey: Prentice Hall.

Honig, M. & Shamai, N. (1978). Family policy as a field—Israel. In Kamerman, S. B. & Kahn, A. J. *Family policy: Government and families in fourteen countries.* New York: Columbia University Press.

Kadushin, A. (1974). *Child welfare services.* (2nd Ed.). New York: Macmillan Publishing Co., Inc.

Kamerman, S. B., & Kahn, A. J. (1978). *Family policy: Government and families in fourteen countries.* New York: Columbia University Press.

Kamerman, S. B., & Kahn, A. J. (1981). *Child care, family benefits, and working parents: A study in comparative policy.* New York: Columbia University Press.

Laufer, Z. (1980). Early-age care-risks and hopes. *Society and Welfare,* 189-201 (in Hebrew).

Littauer, C. (1980). Working with families of children in residential treatment. *Child Welfare, 59,* 225-234.

Littner, N. (1975). The importance of the natural parents to the child in placement. *Child Welfare, 54,* 175-181.

Locke, E. A., Shaw, S., Saari, L. M., & Latham, G. P. (1981). Goal setting and task performance 1969-1980. *Psychological Bulletin, 90,* 125-152.

Magnus, A. (1974). Parent involvement in residential treatment programs. *Children Today, 3*(1), 25-27.

Matsusima, J. (1965). Some aspects of defining "success" in residential treatment. *Child Welfare, 44,* 272-277.

Ministry of Labor and Social Affairs, Child and Youth Department. (1977). *Integration of the home community aspects in treatment of children away from home* (Recommendation) (in Hebrew).

Moss, S. Z. (1969). How children feel about being placed away from home. *Children, 13*(4), 153-157.

Simmons, G., Gumpert, J., & Rothman, B. (1973). Natural parents as partners in child care placement. *Social Casework, 54,* 225-231.

Steers, R. M., & Porter, L. W. (1979). *Motivation and work behavior.* (2nd Ed.). New York: McGraw-Hill.

Weiner, A. (1979). *Differential trends in child placement in the land of Israel 1918-1945.* Unpublished doctoral dissertation, Hebrew University, Jerusalem (in Hebrew).

Wilkes, J. R. (1980). Separation can be a therapeutic option. *Child Welfare, 59,* 27-31.

Williams, J. C. (1972). Helping parents to help their children in placement. *Child Welfare, 51,* 297-303.

Wood, E. P. (1981). Residential treatment for families of maltreated children. *Child Welfare, 60,* 105-108.

Social Conditions
and Pupils' Responses in Israeli
Residential Schools

Yitzhak Kashti
Mordecai Arieli

ABSTRACT. The structure and internal dynamics of Israeli residential schools and change processes that have developed in these settings in recent decades are described. On this basis, parallels and convergences between the institution and the community become apparent, and it is concluded that the residential schools reflect the larger community outside and provide a "second chance" for many of their students to learn to function effectively yet autonomously in that context.

In Israel, the placement of children and adolescents in residential settings is most frequently considered for educational rather than treatment or custodial reasons, especially for disadvantaged young people from the development towns for newer immigrants and the poor districts of the larger cities. Residential programs for such youth provide both a temporary separation from the home and neighbourhood and intensive exposure to the total life situation in the residential setting. Many community officials as well as professionals believe that these two processes tend to reduce possible conflicts between the home community and the educationally enhancing milieu in the setting. They believe that the elimination of such conflicts provides a second chance for the educationally failing pupil, the results of which contribute to successful participation in the Israeli social system and upward social mobility. Largely as a result,

Yitzhak Kashti and Mordecai Arieli are at the School of Education, Tel Aviv University, P.O.B. 39040, Ramat Aviv, Tel Aviv 69978, Israel.

about 18% of Jewish youth in Israel between the ages of 13 and 17 are educated in residential schools.[1]

Although low-achieving, actual and potential dropouts are frequently referred to these settings, some residential schools have become a focus of attraction for the more successful pupils in poorer areas because they serve many middle class students as well and offer prestigious vocational courses; thus, they are viewed as providing a route to social success. This is viewed with semi-ambivalence by community and educational officials. On one hand, the residential schools provide a nonstigmatizing means to serve actual and potential drop-outs and reduce the need to introduce new low-level classes and educational frameworks. On the other hand, the residential schools and the placement authorities are perceived as rival settings competing for the small groups of high achievers (Kashti & Arieli, 1978).[2]

The historical roots of these programs in Israel have been reviewed in the present volume (Weiner, 1985) and elsewhere (e.g., Arieli, Kashti, & Shlasky, 1983). In the 1950s, many new residential schools adopted the bureaucratic structure and formal division into sub-systems of the traditional agricultural schools. From the kibbutz youth group tradition, they took the view that work and social life are educational factors as important as theoretical studies, and the preference for "classic" subject matter as superior to "pragmatic" material. The staff was, as in earlier years, frequently viewed as serving largely as socialization agents. More drastic changes occurred in the 1960s and 1970s, however, at least partly reflecting and in response to changes in the broader society and in the population being served.

For example, relationships between residential schools and neighboring kibbutzim began to weaken, as fewer kibbutz members worked in the schools and the schools trained their students increas-

---

1. For example, the U.S.S.R. has 2% of its total school population in residential school, and England and Wales have 1.9% (Lambert et al., 1975).

2. The reserved attitude of local authorities towards educating their higher achievers in residential settings is reflected, for example, in the two following cases: (1) The "Education Forum" of the Or Yehuda Local Council decided in 1976 to "reexamine the existing policy of sending away gifted children from the town to national or neighbouring institutions"; and (2) During 1977-78 the Local Authority of the township of Hatzor stopped the activities of Youth Aliyah screening and placement officials in the town because they were recruiting relatively high achieving children for residential schools outside the town. Source: correspondence between the Hatzor Local Authority and Youth Aliyah's Executive, Youth Aliyah Archives, 1977-1978.

ingly on their own farms rather than in the kibbutzim. Growing urban areas, on the other hand, often led to closer linkages with neighboring residential schools, which added day programs for town residents and integrated more fully with the community's educational services. Due to declining numbers of immigrants, Youth Aliyah, the largest residential school placement agency, began at least by the early 1970s to focus its attention on placement for non-immigrant youth in educational, social, or financial distress. The concentration of disadvantaged youth in the residential schools was accelerated by sharp cost increases in the 1960s, putting these programs beyond the means of middle class parents who did not seek or qualify for support through public funds. Finally, the emphasis on this approach for the disadvantaged has been supported by the assumption inherent in the Israeli educational system that what are viewed as their cognitive and personality deficits are reversible and can be corrected even in adolescence.

Given the close interaction between the residential school and the community, it seems useful to ask what the structure and the system of the former, viewed as a microcosm, can teach us about the latter and its influence on the development of young people, and this is the focus of the remainder of the paper. Four structural sub-systems are examined first, followed by a section on organizational change and one of the implications for the community.

THE STRUCTURAL SUB-SYSTEMS

Residential schools in Israel generally have at least 140 pupils and 35 full-time staff members; the largest number, together with their day pupils, some 1200 pupils and about 300 staff. In 1979-80, most of the residential schools numbered 200-450 pupils and 50-115 staff. The five key sub-systems are examined here, including: Management, Communication, Control; Residential-Social; Occupational; Schooling; and Treatment.

Management, Communication, Control

Management. The establishment of the residential schools in the early years of the State and in the pre-State period was perceived as part of the process of forming a new society. Therefore, the role of the Principal, who was generally also the founder of the school and often a fairly central member of his political movement, was perceived as one of leadership rather than of "directorship." The Principals were generally not appointed to their posts on the basis of formal professional credentials and through formal procedures such as public tenders, and most created and defined their positions during the process of the school's development rather than entering into a role whose norms were laid down in advance.

Most of the residential schools were quite small (up to 200 pupils). The Principal was directly involved in all the sub-systems, having taken an active part in their establishment. The small size of the programs facilitated this, as did the fact that the Principal was practically the sole liaison between the residential school and the ownership, supervision, and placement agencies.

The founder-Principals gradually reached retirement age. In 1978-79, the majority of Principals of Israeli residential schools had succeeded a previous Principal and came from other positions in the educational system. Without the challenge of creating something new, the new Principals seem to have lost a great deal of the leadership charisma. The development of a tradition more or less common to the residential schools, together with the growing institutionalization of the national educational system and its demands, appear to limit the Principal's opportunity to develop an independent and individual style of management.

In recent years the pattern of the Principal's role has changed as well, as the system he heads becomes increasingly decentralized. One of his main tasks now is to coordinate the various sub-systems, that is, to prevent the over-compartmentalization (or even the disintegration) of the residential school into separate units, and to address the conflicts between the various sub-systems in the light of overall program needs and objectives.

In addition, the Principal still serves as a central figure in safeguarding resources and creating conditions for the school to adjust to its environment, in communicating the goals of the sponsor to the system, in adopting new aims, and in managing a system of communication and control that will guarantee a certain degree of consensus for his and the sponsor's preferred aims.

Communication and Control. The most common formal communication channel in the residential school is the meeting, usually an executive committee meeting or the staff meeting of one of the sub-systems. Generally there is also a great deal of informal communication among the staff in the residential school arising from the fact that they tend to spend a large part of their time together on and off the job. This results from the fact that some staff usually live on grounds, and the roles require staff members who deal with the same child or group of children to be in contact with each other. Informal communication is also intensified in the framework of frequent social gatherings that take place among resident staff members, particularly "metaplot" (housemothers) and "Madrichim" (housefathers). It seems that in most of the residential schools the Principals and the heads of the sub-systems encourage direct approaches to themselves without going through the hierarchy, and such approaches are not generally regarded as bypassing authority.

External control is exercised by the placement and supervision agencies and by the pupils and their parents. In addition, in the residential school, as in every social organization, there is internal control on the part of those in high positions over those in lower positions. Since the residential school may be characterized as an organization with cultural aims, internal control is generally of normative character. In other words, the loyalty of the staff, particularly the educational staff, is apparently based primarily on their identification with the values of the school.

However, it appears that difficulties typical of those existing with regard to the supervision of any educational organization are particularly evident in the residential schools. First, in the absence of defined and clearly measurable student outcomes, criteria of effectiveness of the program, particularly in the living group, tend to be highly diffuse. Second, most of the contacts between the educational staff and the pupils occur in places not easily observed (e.g., the group clubroom, the pupils' dormitory); as in every people-processing organization, it appears that the very presence of the observer, such as the Principal or the head of a department, tends to change the character of the interaction between educational worker and the pupil. Third, it is difficult to control decisions taken in unplanned and unquantifiable situations. Finally, the options for tangibly rewarding or sanctioning residential school staff members are limited, since the staff's relations with the organization are based on work agreements which determine precise, rigid norms of grading and salaries.

The Residential-Social Sub-System

During the hours which are not devoted to schooling or to work, the pupil lives in the framework of the residential-social sub-system. This sub-system, which is headed by the chief "madrich" (the formal head), the chief "metapelet," and the "madrichim" and metaplot (plural for housemothers and housefathers respectively), relates to the pupils' social, leisure, and extra-curricular learning activities. Besides functioning as a formal system, the residential social sub-system serves as the main (if not the only) framework for the activities of the pupils' informal system.

Formal Aspects of the Sub-System. The residential school's pupil population is divided into "youth groups." While most of the students' social interactions take place within these groups, some occur in the frameworks that serve the entire community of students. The residential social sub-system also includes extra-curricular clubs for pupils who are interested in various topics. The youth group consists of 25-70 children of the same age, usually of both sexes. In the special settings for the delinquent or the handicapped the groups are smaller, perhaps as few as 12 or 15 members. Each group has one or two dormitories, which generally include the pupils' rooms, a common room, and (sometimes) an apartment for the "madrich" and/or the "metapelet."

The main formal activity of the youth group is an evening meeting, generally conducted by the "madrich," which takes place 2-3 times a week. Its purposes include: (a) communication and control, organizational coordination, and passing on of information; (b) discussion of current events in Israel and abroad, on subjects of value-idea significance, or on subjects connected with the world of adolescents; (c) parties, games and community singing; and (d) just being together, perhaps watching television, to facilitate cohesion.

The members of the youth group are expected to keep certain rules pertaining to personal and group cleanliness and order, the schedule (e.g., getting up and going to bed), and attendance at group meetings. In addition, the group elects a committee, democratically and with the staff's knowledge, that may introduce additional organizational rules of its own or change existing rules (such as time for lights out), generally after receiving the staff's permission.

In most of the residential schools, all the pupils meet together in the framework of celebrations and ceremonies. A regular and important weekly event is the Sabbath evening ceremony.

Most residential schools also maintain a self-governing body, the central youth council composed of representatives of the youth group committees. The activities of the council, the degree of its independence, the nature of its relations with the management and the staff, and the extent and ways it represents the pupils' interests vary from one residential school to another. The head of the residential-social system operates a network of clubs meeting in the late afternoon for all the pupils in the school. Generally, pupils are obliged to choose one club that meets at least once a week.

Informal Aspects of the Sub-System. Most of the interaction among student peers takes place in the framework of the residential social-informal sub-system. This reflects the fact that in the schooling and the occupational sub-systems, the children are engaged in actions of an individual nature and have a relatively high degree of interaction with adult staff members (teachers and vocational instructors).

Since the members of the youth group spend much of their time together in unstructured dormitory activities, most of the interaction that takes place between them is not formal, and the degree of regular control the adults have over this interaction is limited. The youth group in the residential school acts as a mediating mechanism in permitting dual relations: primary relations between roommates and specific relations with all the members of the peer group in the course of performing shared tasks (Arieli, 1980b).

Roles of the Staff. The Madrich (or housefather) is expected to be at the disposal of his charges during all the daytime hours that are not devoted to formal activity in the schooling or occupational sub-systems, i.e., during mealtimes and in the times set for taking care of their personal belongings, cleaning their dormitories, doing homework, social activities, and leisure. The nature of the pupils' activities during the time they are supervised by the madrich indicates the wide variety of components of his role. These components require a developmental and custodial orientation towards the pupils, and the skill to relate simultaneously to the individual and the group.

According to Goffman (1961), one of the characteristics of the total institution that undermines the inmate's personality is his dependence on a large and complex apparatus in order to satisfy his smallest needs. An educational organization with total characteristics needs, therefore, someone who can help the resident to maintain the integration of his personality. It appears that the general expectation in the residential school until recently was that this task would be done by the madrich. However, the madrich is expected to perform additional functions which may be classified as (1) individual-developmental functions; (2) group developmental functions; (3) individual custodial functions; and (4) group custodial functions.

During the 1930s and 1940s, the social component of the role of the madrich was considered the major one; the madrich was perceived as the central factor in recruiting the pupils to the ideology of agricultural settlement. In the fifties and sixties, when the politically "ideological" education systems were replaced by the State education system with its strong achievement orientation together with increasing concern for the child's individual well-being, the individual component of the madrich's role appears to have been increasingly emphasized over the social component. This emphasis was reflected in the large amount of time devoted by the madrich to helping with homework and to other, individual supportive talks.

Since the mid-seventies, another change in the role of the madrich has occurred. Helping with homework is gradually being taken out of his hands, because he is neither equipped with knowledge of the subject matter taught in the secondary school, nor trained in the didactic techniques required for helping pupils with learning problems. Instead, many residential schools have developed study groups run by specialists who are not regular members of the school staff. As a result, the individual pupil joins in many extra-group activities, thus reducing the extent of his direct contact with the madrich. This process has increased with the introduction of clinical school psychologists, educational counsellors, social workers, and other specialists who are expected to provide a large amount of the support for which students previously looked to the madrich.

This state of affairs makes the madrich largely a supervisor of the pupils' participation in the various activities and an agent of discipline. The increasingly custodial nature of the role is sometimes explained by the madrichim themselves as a response to the growing tendency of the pupils from disadvantaged groups to reject the school's management and to regard the madrich as an agent thereof. However, the changed emphasis in the role of the madrich has not changed his role prescriptions; the impression is that the madrich is still expected to fulfill simultaneously individual and social, custodial and developmental functions despite the inherent conflicts between them.

The metapelet (or housemother) complements the madrich in charge of one of the educational groups in the residential school. The metapelet's role prescriptions include caring for the personal cleanliness of the group members, the cleanliness and tidiness of their rooms, their health and clothing, their eating habits and nourishment, and also their general feeling of well-being. The metaplot eat lunch with their pupils and in some residential schools supervise or help with the serving of food. When the group members return to the dormitory the metaplot have personal talks with the pupils, particularly those in the younger age groups and apparently particularly with the girls in these groups. The metapelet's role prescriptions and work schedule show that she is required to respond to two groups of needs of the pupils; adaptive needs and tension-release needs. The desire to meet these two types of needs through one role-bearer is drawn from the model of the family: The metapelet is perceived as the mother of the group.

In order to respond to these two groups of needs, two basic concepts of the metapelet's role have emerged, particularly in the last decade: the service-custodial approach and the formative-development approach. The service-custodial approach is expressed in role components such as keeping order, maintaining cleanliness and following the schedule. The formative-developmental approach is expressed in such components as caring for the well-being and comfort of the pupils and having supportive talks with individuals. These two perspectives emphasize the diffuse, obscure, and often conflicting aspects of the metapelet's role. The conflict between the custodial and the formative aspects of the metapelet's role appears to be particularly pressing since the custodial aspects are overt and convenient for definition, expectation, and reward, while the formative role components exist mainly as an approach and not as definitions of performance.

While madrichim are mostly young men in their twenties and the average duration of their employment is about two years, the ages of the metaplot vary widely and the average duration of their employment is about fifteen years. Thus, they are frequently many years older than the madrichim and the students with whom they work; this is regarded as a problem by many of the older metaplot.

The Occupational Sub-System

Until the mid-1950s, the programs of most residential schools in Israel, including those not defined as agricultural schools, included working on a farm maintained on the school grounds or nearby. Work in general, and agricultural work in particular, were perceived as vital for the preparation of young people for a pioneering life in the framework of rural settlement and as a way of national social regeneration. Training in agricultural work was, therefore, considered to be an integral part of the formal school curriculum.

Beginning in the mid-fifties, however, the status of the farm and agricultural training in about 70% of the residential schools began to change in two directions. Some decided to turn their institutions into vocational or academic secondary schools, or into comprehensive schools containing both academic and vocational tracks, while others decided to preserve the agricultural character of the school but introduced courses in agromechanics for all or some of the pupils alongside the traditional agricultural studies. In both cases, the changes were explained as a response to the accelerated industrialization and urbanization in Israel and to the requests of the pupils and their parents for a curriculum designed to prepare students for roles in an industrialized urban society or for a general matriculation certificate leading to university admission.

In the vocationally-oriented schools, several hours a day are typically devoted to practical training in the various technical subjects studied by the pupils; this training does not seem to be generally perceived by the pupils and staff as work, but as an essential part of learning the subject. The general tendency in residential schools that are not agricultural is, however, to engage all the pupils in various services, particularly in the dining-room, gardening and grounds work, and guard duty. Having the pupils occupied in services appears to have additional implications in two ways: economizing on the need for hired adult labor; and custodial significance, or as one of the Principals put it: "Organized employment prevents idleness, thus preventing delinquent behavior."

In the agriculturally focused residential schools, a separate subsystem deals with the employment of pupils. The function of this sub-system is to run the farm, whose formal status is equal to that of the schooling and residential social sub-systems. Generally the tendency is to employ the pupils in most of the agricultural and vocational branches and also in facility services during their first two years of the four-year course. This appears to be a relic of the approach that prevailed in the kibbutzim during the British Mandate, of employing the members on a rotation system which allows the pupils to experience many kinds of work and to choose one or two in which to specialize during the next two years. About 70% of the third-year pupils in the agricultural schools specialize in one of the farm branches in their third year, and approximately half of all the pupils work regularly in the branch they have chosen for specialization during their last two years at the school.

The Schooling Sub-System

The schooling sub-system resembles a day school in its aims and structure; it is often called "the school" in the context of the institution itself, which is viewed as a whole from the outside as a residential school. Indeed, this "school within a school" operates as a 4-year secondary school, or as a 6-year school comprising a Middle and Upper School.

The academic level of the schools is not uniform: technical skills are taught at a very low level of sophistication in some, while the standard is considered to be very high relative to Israeli secondary schools as a whole in others. Some offer only one specialization (agricultural or maritime), while others are comprehensive and offer three or more courses at three levels. The schools function during the morning and early afternoon, for 36 to 42 weeks per year.

With the establishment of a central State education system that superceded the schools operated by the political parties, the Ministry of Education began to define the formal curricula, including those of the residential schools. Also, the Ministry of Education, through its various departments, began to supervise the level of teaching and the scholastic achievements. Changes in the formal curriculum were apparently a response to the growing interest of many pupils and parents in studies leading to a vocation in an industrialized urban society or providing general education and a certificate (matriculation) permitting university entrance. From the late fifties on, many Principals and educators in residential schools began to report an increase in the status of educational studies among the pupils, relative to their interest in "social life" and work.

The independence of the residential schooling sub-system increased when local youth began to be admitted as day students in the late fifties. Since the day students' dependence on the residential school's other sub-systems was minimal, their entrance into the school led to a growth in the strength and autonomy of the schooling sub-system.

Teachers in the residential schools require the same training as those in day secondary schools. Most earned a first degree at a university in one or two subjects and were subsequently trained as teachers of those subjects. Until the early fifties, many teachers acted in a combined role of teacher and madrich. This combination, which had its origin in the tradition of the kibbutz youth group, brought the teacher-madrich to educational activity of an expressive social character alongside the instrumental teaching activity. With increased differentiation in the structure of the residential school, the total number of educational workers acting as a teacher-madrich decreased, but there are still teachers who received university training for teaching roles while working as madrichim.

The Treatment Sub-System

From the time they were established, the residential schools in Israel were perceived as educational settings rather than child care institutions. The pupils were perceived as ordinary children who had to be educated and to learn certain social values and norms. The staff members were perceived as educators, that is, adults whose role was to perform the functions of teaching the children and inculcating in them the values and norms of the culture. In contrast to child care institutions, youth in the residential schools were not considered deviant and in need of rehabilitation, treatment, or resocialization, and the majority of the staff members were not treatment professionals.

In recent years, apparently as a result of growing awareness on the part of the residential schools and placement agencies concerning the possibilities opened by the treatment professions for treating youths with a background of social distress, small treatment sub-systems have developed in some of the residential schools. These sub-systems include 1-4 workers, with multiple professional backgrounds: educational counselors, social workers, and clinical school psychologists. They function primarily as consultants to the educational staff and in treating individual pupils.

Consultation to the Educational Staff. The treatment worker is expected to maintain contacts with the educational staff, particularly the madrichim and metaplot. At meetings, the educational worker is expected to bring up his concerns in working with the pupils as a group or as individuals, or problems concerning his relations with his colleagues on the staff, while the treatment worker is expected to respond by advising on and helping him to work through the various dilemmas.

Many educational workers are reluctant to have treatment personnel in the residential school, however, since they see the entrance of the individual worker with his esoteric knowledge and the prestige this knowledge carries as endangering their status and with it their influence on the management and on students. Further, educational workers, who are exposed to constant and diffuse contact with pupils, tend sometimes to view the short time spent by the treatment worker with difficult students as an expression of limited involvement with the students and their problems and as unwillingness to devote themselves fully to the task of solving such problems. The primary barrier to the role of the treatment worker as a consultant is, therefore, the tendency of some of the educational staff to avoid contact and cooperation with him.

Treatment of Pupils. The treatment worker is expected to help individual students to work out their personal and social problems. In some residential schools, there are established procedures to help individuals to approach the treatment worker on their own initiative. However, the pupils who are under the care of the treatment worker are generally those referred by the educational staff because of behavior perceived as deviant or troublesome. Further, since the treatment worker concentrates on the personality and motives of the individual, treatment is perceived by the educational staff and the management of the residential school as a process that tends to legitimize the failure to achieve norms, that is, as a process opposed to the educational goals.

ORGANIZATIONAL CHANGE AND PUPILS' RESPONSE

Various studies and observations seem to indicate that residential schools have undergone a process of change during the last three decades, a process of similar directions but different levels of intensity in each school (Kashti & Arieli, 1977). The change can be summed up as involving: (a) a decrease in level of ideological closedness; (b) the shifting of the guiding social orientation from status to role preparation; (c) an increase in the importance that staffs attribute to instrumental aims; (d) decentralization of organizational structure; (e) increase in staff role differentiation; and (f) increase in centrality of professional affiliation as an occupation frame of reference for many staff members.

A. A decrease in level of ideological closedness. The principals of ideologically "closed" schools have gradually reduced the tendency to recruit their junior staff members from among individuals who are ideologically committed to either the general ethos of pioneering or, more specifically, to the movements which own the settings. Principals of party-owned schools and their management committees have "opened" their settings and have begun to recruit heads of important sub-systems, such as the schooling and the residential sub-systems, from among professionals who are not identified with the party.

B. *The shifting of the guiding social orientation from status to role preparation.* Until the early 1950s, the educational programs focused on extending the range of the socializing process to the overall status of the pupil, and in a broad and integrative manner to develop his self-perception beyond his specific future roles. More recently, however, the programs have tended, in varying degrees, to limit the influence of the socialization process to training for differentiated and specific roles in the adult society in which the students are expected to participate.

C. *An increase in the importance that staffs attribute to instrumental aims.* Until the early 1950s, expressive goals were considered primary or at least equal in importance to instrumental goals, both at the stated and implemented levels. This meant, for example, that the financial resources allotted to extracurricular activities and the prestige of the madrichim were not significantly lower than the resources allotted to schooling and the prestige of the teachers. At present, it seems that the latent message transmitted by the senior to the junior staff and to the pupils is that schooling and schoolmasters are more highly valued than social activities and madrichim.

D. *Decentralization of organizational structure.* In the early 1950s the schools were characterized by a centralized pattern of organization, as reflected in the nature of their internal and external organizational relations. The school's decisions tended to be made by the principal who, as he saw fit, delegated certain executive power to the heads of the sub-systems, and they to their deputies, according to a hierarchical pattern. The school's relations with the outside world were also largely initiated and regulated by the principal, who served as the almost exclusive agent and transmitter of the norms and expectations of the external systems to all ranks of the school. Since the late 1950s these centralized features have been replaced by decentralized ones. The changes are reflected in the structure of internal relations within the staff, which now tend to be characterized by a fairly high level of autonomy of the heads of the sub-systems as regards policy of their units, relative freedom of decision allowed to low-ranking members of the staff, and the status—of coordinator of more or less autonomous sub-systems— assigned to the principal. The school's relations with external agencies tend to be based on the autonomy of the heads of the sub-systems in maintaining direct relationships with role partners outside the system.

E. Increase in staff role differentiation. In the early 1950s the areas of activity and the roles of the staff in all the schools were not highly differentiated and were often even diffuse or interchangeable. In many cases, the educator—a role combining formal and informal functions—acted as both schoolmaster and madrich. More recently, the relations of staff members with the students have become relatively differentiated. This is reflected, among other things, in the fact that these relations have become largely delineated by the specific skill and the definition of the staff member's role.

F. Increase in centrality of professional affiliation as an occupation frame of reference for many staff members. In the 1950s most teachers at the residential schools tended to consider the organization in which they worked as their most significant occupational frame of reference. This was probably partly due to the fact that teachers tended to live in the setting, and partly due to their relative lack of qualifications. At present, most teachers, counselors (madrichim), and social workers in the residential schools seem to attribute more significance to their professional identity than to their organizational affiliation. In general, teachers, counselors, and social workers are now more qualified and live outside the school campus.

The six dimensions of change offered here can be described as six aspects of movement along a continuum from "closedness" to "openness." The following diagram expresses graphically the positions that Israeli residential schools in general seem to have held on these continua in 1950, two years after the emergence of the State of Israel, and in the 1970s.

The Open Model—1970s		The Closed Model—1950s
ideological openness	_____	ideological closeness
role socialization	_____	status socialization
centrality of instrumental goals	_____	centrality of expressive roles
decentralization	_____	centralization
differentiated staff roles	_____	diffuse staff roles
professional norms	_____	organizational norms

It will be recalled that, in the first years of the State, the residential school largely took the place of the kibbutz youth group of the

1930s and 1940s and acquired some of its characteristics. The staff members' commitment to the agricultural and pioneering ideology as a super-ordinate goal continued to give residential education an elitist character on the pattern of the classic kibbutz youth group. In this situation, the pupils tended to identify with their educators and to intenalize their social concepts. Various observations lead us to assume that the reduced commitment of the staff members to any super-ordinate goal led—at least partly—to reduced identification of the students with the staff and their social goals. Thus, there was an increased need to create an alternative system which would provide objects for student loyalty.

Education for settling on the land continued to characterize the youth village in the early years of the State. By its very nature, such education tended to avoid training the pupils in specific skills or for professional diplomas and stressed "general education," or "education of the person." The status socialization of the "pioneer" or the "settler" entailed a lifestyle which encompassed every aspect of the pupils' lives: in the classroom, at work, and in social activities. Thus, it was internally consistent and limited the possibilities of internal conflicts. As the residential schools shifted from status socialization to role socialization, namely, training pupils in specific skills, and as the unifying themes receded, it appears that students have sought alternative or supplementary social frameworks offering compensating cohesion.

The growing importance of preparing the individual for a career, a diploma, and a profession limited students' opportunities to engage in expressive activities. The formal status of the madrich, who is responsible for activities of a tension-relieving nature, declined as his traditional social and ideological function was to some extent pushed aside. It may also be that as expressive activity loses status in the formal system, students resort to an alternative system permitting these activities in an informal manner.

As the staff members' commitment to a unifying social theme decreases, and with the growing importance of instrumental training for differential roles, the centralized organizational pattern of a setting tends often to be replaced by a decentralized pattern. Hence, the residential school gradually ceases to provide the students with a cohesive organization having coordinated expectations. The decentralization of the organization in itself also adds to the need for an alternative or supplementary system based on the peer group.

The more that education tends to take on an instrumental character, and the more differentiated its goals become, the greater seems to be the need for staff members with specific specializations. The professional with a specific, perhaps esoteric, specialization tends to restrict his contacts with the pupils to the area in which he is training them, a process which denies the pupil diffuse interaction with significant adults holding status—the power structure of the organization.

The growing role differentiation of some of the staff members, particularly the teachers, also seems related to the diminished status of the setting as their occupational frame of reference. The sources of their role norms are outside the residential school, in the disciplines they specialized in, the universities where they studied, and the professional associations to which they belong or hope to belong. With the increased importance of the professional frame of reference for the staff member, his solidarity with the organization seems to decrease. He is no longer a "local" group leader, but a "cosmopolitan" professional who chances to be in a bureaucratic organization. Perhaps the pupils' informal system, which provides leaders for the peer group, is designed to compensate also for the loss in leaders from the setting's formal system.

It appears that the more "open" the residential schools are, the more the pupils tend to feel frustration and lack of identification, leading to the creation of a compensatory and supplementary informal system which rejects the unsatisfactory, formal system. This attitude of the pupils may be explained, at least partly, as a reaction to the changes in the structure of the residential schools. In those residential schools where there is least commitment on the part of the staff members to an ideology, where the emphasis is on socialization for differential roles and instrumental aims, where the organizational pattern is decentralized, where many of the staff perform differentiated functions and regard their professional affiliation as their central occupational frame of reference, the pupils seem to feel abandoned by the adult.

The impact of the residential school on the affective and social development of disadvantaged adolescents tends to be positive, as evidenced in several studies (Kashti, 1974; Feuerstein et al., 1976; Kashti, 1979; Smilansky & Nevo, 1979). However, observations suggest that the residential school pupil is more or less prepared for what he is coming to, on the basis of information gleaned from parents, older siblings, and friends who have spent some time in residential settings (Arieli, 1980a). It is doubtful whether he feels any anxiety about the "closed" and structured world of the residential school, an image prevalent in literature on residential settings. His prior judgements are fairly clear with regard to some of the people and domains he is about to meet, and with regard to others he does not hesitate to change his attitudes, particularly in the direction of limiting the setting's nearness to him, and perhaps even its influence on him. He tends to reject the "totality" of the institution, to the extent that this exists. He is not an easy object to be swallowed up in the culture of the setting; he is not an easy object for acts of cultural colonization or co-optation. He does not regard the setting as his home, nor the metaplot and madrichim as substitute parents; nor does he expect the teachers to bring about sweeping changes in his schooling career or his social standing.

The observations tend further to indicate that the student's motives in setting his priorities for the residential school experience derive from his expectations for the future and his preparation for it, and are often formed before entering the residential setting. Perhaps the residential school helps to consolidate his motives and expectations, and it obviously helps him to prepare himself for his future role, but only rarely does it tend to instill in him these motives and expectations or to form them. In other words, before entering the residential school, the students have been socialized towards support or rejection of a large number of "items" in that new setting. This pre- or anticipatory socialization is apparently the main key to the understanding of students' priorities.

Most residential school students do not appear to be seeking highly structured relationships or organizational forms and authority, particularly when these are associated with adult figures. They understand and appreciate order and discipline, but they do not want these to be forced on them in a patronizing manner. Observations show that with the passage of time, students tend to open up to members of their peer group. The formal "Youth Group" in the residential setting—that "historical entity" which has been the subject of changing rationales throughout the years and is today regarded by youth village educators as a solution to many of the problems of the individual and the society, a strong source of support and resocialization—this formal group does not, however, seem to arouse students to the anticipated involvement and identification.

It seems that the pupil's career leads in the direction of instrumental goals. He "knows" that he has to be orderly and observe the rules, he knows the value of good friends and informal involvement in his peers' lives, he knows that he has to study and be active in learning, and he has learned, in the course of his time at the residential school, that work can be a thing of value, and even interesting and satisfying. The oft-stated advantage of the residential setting on the educational level—that is, the possibility of setting and realizing expressive goals of a quality and scope largely unattainable in other socialization settings does not find expression in recent studies.

It seems clear that we do not have here the subdued inmates of a total institution, nor young members of the elite being co-opted to their school culture, leading them smoothly (or roughly) to the status of prominent civil servants and pioneers. We have here a setting which is largely a reflection of daily life as it is perceived by its disadvantaged pupils, although it maintains some of the features of its tradition. The students often circumvent these "historical strongholds" in various ways. The traditional impact of this socialization setting, particularly in the ideological and expressive domains, appears to have been dissipated, and its pupils draw from it mainly what they had wanted before they arrived. Thus, the residential school seems to emerge as primarily a framework for a second chance for those whose chances tend to be limited. And they seem frequently to make good use of it to meet their needs in the way they themselves understand and define them.

REFERENCES

Arieli, M. (1980a). The peer group in the residential setting: Some of the features of its informal system. In S. Adiel, H. Shalom, & M. Arieli (Eds.), *Fostering deprived youth and residential education* (pp. 327-337). Tel Aviv: Tcherikover (in Hebrew).

Arieli, M. (1980b). *The role of disadvantaged pupils in Israeli residential schools.* Unpublished doctoral dissertation, The University of Sussex, England.

Arieli, M., Kashti, Y., & Shlasky, S. (1983). *Living at school: Israeli residential schools as people processing organizations.* Tel-Aviv: Ramot Pub. Co., Research Notebooks No. 1.

Feuerstein, R., Hoffman, N., Krasilowski, D., Rand, Y., & Tannenbaum, A. J. (1976). The effects of group care on the psychosocial habilitation of immigrant adolescents in Israel with special reference to high-risk children. *International Review of Applied Psychology, 25,* 189-201.

Goffman, E. (1961). *Asylums.* New York: Doubleday.

Kashti, Y. (1974). *Socially disadvantaged youth in residential education in Israel.* Unpublished doctoral dissertation. The University of Sussex, England.

Kashti, Y. (1979). *The socializing community: Disadvantaged adolescents in Israeli youth villages.* (SEE Monograph Series No. 1) Tel Aviv: Tel Aviv University.

Kashti, Y., & Arieli, M. (1977). Toward a classification of residential settings. In D. Nevo (Ed.), *Theory and research in educational practice.* Tel Aviv: Tel Aviv University (in Hebrew).

Kashti, Y., & Arieli, M. (Eds.). (1978). *The supportive system: An experiment in developing community education systems.* Tel Aviv: Tel Aviv University (in Hebrew).

Lambert, R., Bullock, R., & Millham, S. (1975). *The chance of a lifetime? A study of boys' and coeducational boarding schools in England and Wales.* London: Weidenfeld & Nicholson.

Smilansky, M., & Nevo, D. (1979). *The gifted disadvantaged: A ten year longitudinal study of compensatory education in Israel.* New York and London: Gordon and Breach.

Weiner, A. (1985). Institutionalizing institutionalization: The historical roots of residential care in Israel. *Child & Youth Services, 7*(3/4), pp 3-19.

Institution as Community

Yochanan Wozner

ABSTRACT. Seven variables basic to the idea of "community" are examined in relation to the organization of institutions: status, role definition, mobility, unifying theme, sanction system, communication, and decision making. It is argued that not all characteristics of the traditional community are helpful for understanding the organization of institutions, and that the unifying theme is the major independent variable which influences the development of an effective institution. If a unifying theme does not exist, then open communication, a dispersed decision-making process, and a graded sanction system may help to fill the void.

The focus of this paper is on organizational aspects of out-of-home care for people who society wishes to reclaim to its ranks by temporary or permanent institutional group care. Such out-of-home care is usually provided by such agencies as boarding schools, residential treatment centers, hospitals, prisons, etc. I use a generic name for these organizations: "internats" (Wozner, 1972; Wolins & Wozner, 1977, 1982). Group home and family foster care arrangements are not explicitly included, although some of what follows is relevant to such settings as well.

INTEGRATED RECLAIMING INTERNATS

Internats are said to perform an integrative function for society (Parsons, 1956), but this function may be performed without regard for the needs of the individuals involved. Internats which segregate and warehouse people may fulfill a socially integrative function (social reclaiming), but they do not reclaim the individuals living there (personal reclaiming). Only internats which attempt to change inmates in a way which enables them to join the larger society as

Yochanan Wozner, School of Social Work, Tel Aviv University, P.O.B. 39040, Ramat Aviv, Tel Aviv 69978, Israel.

full-fledged members, whether after they leave the internat or while they are in it, can be considered as *integrated reclaiming internats.* That is, these internats work to integrate the needs of society and the needs of the inmate in the reclaiming process (Wolins & Wozner, 1982). They include, for example, many boarding schools, British "public schools," and Israeli youth villages whose objective is to prepare the inmates for participation in society after they leave the internats. Similarly, the better homes for the aged and internats for the physically handicapped, which enable their residents to participate significantly in the outside world while enabling them to meet the special needs resulting from each individual's particular impediment, accomplish integrated reclaiming.

The Social Context of Integrated Reclaiming

An integrated reclaiming internat can exist only in a societal context where there is no overriding qualitative differentiation between individuals or groups. If a society views some of its members as fundamentally different in ways that are unchangeable, then social and personal reclaiming are irreconcilable. If some individuals or groups are viewed as having more limited rights than others, then integrated reclaiming is seldom attempted for the deprived. Thus, my assumption is that integrated reclaiming internats can be organized only for those members of society who are considered to be potential full partners in its social context and, *ipso facto,* only in societies which view their members as potentially equal. The more pluralistic a society, the fewer individuals or groups will be excluded from the integrated reclaiming process.

Paradoxically, however, the more pluralistic a society, the less prone will it be to tolerate internat living for some of its members. When, as in pluralistic societies, avenues of mobility are many and open for almost all, the importance of ascribed or inherited status is formally minimized; where the changeability (development) of people is taken for granted, there is normally also a strong demand for the abolition of internat care. This would not present a major problem if alternative arrangements for those who have no place to live or who cannot now be cared for adequately in the community would be forthcoming. However, such arrangements do not seem to be widely available. Alternatives to institutions have helped to differentiate between populations and types of internats but have not yet demonstrated that internat care can be dismissed or that there is no need to seek ways to modify and improve existing internat arrangements. Thus it seems to be justified to continue and even to intensify efforts to develop more effective internat organization. My point of departure is that internats are legitimate and normative social institutions and, therefore, I seek ways of increasing their capacity for integrated reclaiming.

TOWARD IMPROVING INTERNATS

One approach to improving the integrated reclaiming ability of the internat is to delimit its bureaucratic structuring and to encourage the movement toward a more community-like organization, which involves two major dimensions. The first concerns the relationship of the internat as an entity to its environment, the community. In this regard, it has been suggested above that societal attitude toward the internat and the activity within is of cardinal importance for the implementation of integrated reclaiming. It seems to be absolutely necessary that differentiated, bilateral transactions should exist between the environment and the internat, lest the internat and its members (staff and clients alike) stagnate (Wolins & Wozner, 1982).

The second dimension concerns the internat's internal organization. This has been addressed by many practitioners who have tried to approximate what they regarded as optimal community arrangements. Salzman (1785, 1869), for example, organized *Schnepfenthal,* a residential school founded in 1784 as a community of "families" in which the inmates were under the care of the "head of the family." The program emphasized the study of the local environment, farming, carpentry, mining, industry, etc. The children participated in running the internat by fulfilling a variety of "public positions." They could earn by performing special tasks and were independent in deciding how to spend their savings. There was an elaborate reward-punishment system, differentiated by age. Achievement was well rewarded; for example, Salzman's daughter at the age of 14 became a member of the "Order of Diligence," an achieved status, and started to teach younger children. An elaborate point system governed entry to this order.

Schnepfenthal is not the only example of attempts to "communitize" internats; similar experiments are reported by many (see, for example, George & Stoew, 1912; Lane, 1913; Simpson, 1916; Badley, 1937; Bazeley, 1948; Makarenko, 1955; Reinhold, 1953; Super, 1957; Bentwich, 1960; Wolins & Gottesmann, 1971; Porat, 1977; Golan, 1977). The major common element evident in these efforts is the desire to heighten the participation of the internat's residents in the reclaiming process by some idiosyncratic arrangement which makes the internat more community-like. This tendency has also influenced internats for the mentally ill (Jones, 1953; Fairweather, 1964). The strategies adopted to accomplish this feat range from the guided permissiveness of Summerhill (Neill, 1960) to the carefully structured group arrangement of Fairweather et al. (1969). In any case the notion that a community-like internat is the better internat seems to be well established. But then what is a community?

INTERNAT AS COMMUNITY

The term community has many meanings. Hillery (1955), reviewing 94 definitions of community, concludes that, "there is one element, however, which can be found in all of the concepts, . . . all of the definitions deal with people. Beyond this common basis, there is no agreement" (p. 117). What, then, do we mean when we think of the internat as community? Hillery's comment assures us that at least we are talking about some arrangement which concerns people, and internats are organizations which also deal with people, including as clients those they seek to change. The desired changes may be implicit or declared, specific or diffuse.

Organizers of internats are continually looking for ways to organize them as effectively and, perhaps, as efficiently as possible. Organizers of integrated reclaiming internats seek ways to avoid those attributes of organizations that may enhance the development of non-desired relationships among people or the acceleration of detrimental behavior patterns. One approach is to organize internats as communities. Why is community selected as the model? What are the characteristics of the community which are to be emulated in the internat?

I suggest that the community concept was selected by internat organizers because it helped to "de-institutionalize" the internat as a "total institution," a trend which is widely supported by professionals, and not because community characteristics were found to be directly helpful for integrated reclaiming. Further, some attributes of community imply similarity to the family, which is traditionally accepted to be the natural habitat of the individual and, especially, of children; thus, calling the internat ''community'' may alleviate the dissonance between internat and family. Such considerations may not be entirely faulty, because names and labels influence people's conceptions of reality, but in order to apply attributes of ''community'' more effectively to the organization of reclaiming internats, one has to examine the attributes and select those which best fit the needs of the integrated reclaiming internat.

Community as Gemeinschaft

Tonnies (1957), whose work yielded variables for generations of sociologists studying societies, communities, and organizations, described three kinds of communities:

a. locality, a geographic or spatial community based upon common habitat;
b. ''mind'' communities, meaning the cooperation and coordinated effort of people for a common goal, not necessarily in one locality; and
c. kinship communities, that is, the extended family.

He further distinguished between two major modes of organization: the *Gesellschaft,* characterized by formal and explicit bonds with formally structured relationships and hierarchical authority arrangements; and the *Gemeinschaft* (usually translated as community), characterized by implicit bonds between members. These bonds include common values, mutual interdependence, shared cultural traditions, and similar social expectations. Relationships among members of the Gemeinschaft are intimate and enduring. There is a clear understanding of each person's status and a ''man's worth'' is estimated according to *who* he is, not *what* he has done (Bell & Newby, 1971):

> In a community, roles are specific and consonant with one another: a man does not find his duties in one role conflicting with the duties that devolve upon him from another role. Members of a community are relatively immobile in a physical and a social way: individuals neither travel from their locality of birth nor do they rise up the social hierarchy. In addition, the culture of the community is relatively homogeneous for it must be so if roles are not to conflict or human relations to lose their intimacy. (p. 24)

From this description we can deduce a number of attributes central to the nature of community:

1. Status is ascriptive rather than achieved;
2. Roles are specific rather than different, and there is a minimum of role conflict;
3. There is a low level of mobility, spatially and socially;
4. There is a common value system, prescribing norms of behavior and similar expectations; and
5. Sanctions are allocated not for specific deeds or the lack of them, but for general attitudes (Parsons, 1968).

These attributes will be examined next in the context of the integrated reclaiming purpose of the internat:

Status. The status of the person who is in the internat (differentiated from the status of the internat among other social institutions) may be discussed from two points of view. First, consider the change from the status of being a non-resident to the status of a resident. The nature of this change depends on the type of the internat the person joins. Entering the Military Academy, a leading yeshiva (Jewish talmudical college), or another high prestige internat may shift the status of the new recruit in an upward direction, while entering a correctional institution will probably shift even a previously high status person downwards, except perhaps within the context of a criminal sub-culture. In any case, however, even from this point of view, status change exists and demonstrates that status is to be achieved and not purely ascriptive.

More important, however, is the second perspective, concerning changes in status *within* the internat as a result of the reclaiming process. This is, of course, the heart of the matter. Possibly the most important condition for successful reclaiming is to perceive the residents' status not as ascribed to him, but as temporary and changeable through a given set of activities, which constitute the reclaiming processes of the internat. If illness, mental or physical, retardation, poverty, delinquency, etc., are perceived as only slightly changeable, ascribed status attributes, as is often the case in traditional cultures, then efforts to change such statuses are *a priori* doomed to failure. Thus, if a person's status is determined by who he is and not by what he does, then the resident's performance is of no consequence except in internats "demanding (only) that its wards adjust to the norms of the institution" (Kashti, 1979, p. 20), a demand which does not necessarily lead to integrated reclaiming. Status ascription implies that people change only by *becoming more what they are,* but do not become something that they were not ("second order change") (Watzlawick et al., 1974). But we do not, of course, want the deprived to become more deprived, the retarded more retarded, and the criminal more criminal, etc.; we want "second order change" to occur. Strategies of reclaiming are devised to break down global classifications and emphasize multiple dimensions of capability and incapability so that the resident may progress in different channels toward a more desired and normatively accepted "status" (Wolins & Wozner, 1977).

Roles. Role differentiation within a system is suggested by Wilensky and Lebeaux (1958, pp. 58-63) as a measure of division of labor. Role allocation based on the subdivision of tasks into specialized responsibilities requiring specific skills results in high involvement in performance (Blau et al., 1966). There is a broad spectrum of tasks to be performed in an internat. Thus, specificity of roles, an attribute of the community, would seem to be helpful in the running of an internat.

High specialization may also atomize the contact between people, however, thus creating in the internat a disruption of comprehensive interaction between caretakers and care recipients. In some of the more successful internats, caretaker roles are quite diffuse in terms of their comprehensiveness. This applies, for example, to the "mutti" in the SOS Kinderdorf (Wolins, 1968), and to the "madrich" and the "metapelet" in Israeli youth villages (Shalom, 1980). These roles lend themselves more to diffuse characterization than to precise definition as specific roles, their specialized nature notwithstanding. It is characteristic of these roles that their fulfillment requires *total* responsibility. The "madrich" in a traditional youth village is responsible for the overall, mental, physical and, social well-being of his ward. Thus, the resident knows that he has one "special" person responsible for him and also one person to whom he may turn with any problem he might have. Such specialization is person (resident)-focused as contrasted with "professional specialization," which is problem-oriented. The former is a special person for the resident (a generalist), while the latter is a "specialist" dealing with a specific category of problems. An integrated reclaiming internat is best served by the prevalence of the non-specific but "special-person" type of role allocation.

One internat in Israel with which the author is personally familiar required the accountant to fill in for the cook, the vocational teacher to stay over some weekends to be with the residents, the social worker to teach in the classroom, and the director (occasionally) to clean the sewer (ouch!). This was done to give visibility to the idea that the functioning of the internat is the concern of everyone involved. Although each of us had quite clearly defined areas of responsibility and considerable training to carry them out, it was also understood that the definition of responsibilities did not delimit their scope but, rather, pinpointed their focus. Role diffusion was seen as desirable.

Mobility. Social and physical mobility are restricted in the Gemeinschaft. Everyone knows his place within the social structure and people are discouraged from traveling far from the locality. Both these attributes exist in internats and, when applied totally and literally, both seem to be dysfunctional to the reclaiming effort. Lack of social mobility creates the "binary structure" (staff and "inmates") lamented by many students of internat care (Goffman, 1961; Wheeler, 1966). Restriction of spatial movement interferes with the residents' opportunities to interact with the outside environment. Such an arrangement is obviously not what one would expect from a reclaiming internat, where an important vehicle of change is the opportunity to model people who are considered to represent the kind of "changed person" viewed as desirable. Such modeling incorporates the knowledge and expectation that its successful accomplishment will result in achieving the model's status. Thus, in an integrated reclaiming internat, mobility (social and spatial) should be encouraged and should be an inherent part of its activity. The main channels of mobility should be provided for the residents who are the subject of the reclaiming effort. Staff members should have the opportunity to move from one position to another and both within and beyond the internat; more importantly, they should also be provided with an opportunity to progress personally, a task usually known as staff development.

Common value system. A value system that is shared by the members of the internat is probably one of the most important characteristics for the achievement of the reclaiming goal. Successful reclaiming effort in an internat requires that the internat have "an ideology according to which beliefs about the ongoings within the internat have compatible components, and the performance prescribed by these beliefs in terms of objectives and tasks corresponds to accepted norms within the internat" (Wozner, 1972, p.78). Such ideology or Unifying Theme (Wolins & Wozner, 1977) serves as a "great arbitrator" between conflicting views and idiosyncratic expectations. It is a yardstick for the allocation of sanctions, positive and negative, and provides boundaries for setting goals and verifying their attainment. Such a unifying theme need not be political—it can be "A guiding idea or philosophy, which is understandable to, and providing hope for, all members of the institution. . . ." (Reppucci, 1973, p. 333). A unifying theme is often personified by a charismatic leader (Makarenko, 1955; Korczak, 1967), while in other cases it may be the heritage of some past event or a utopian vision of things to come (Reinhold, 1953; Rinott, 1971).

The centrality of shared values in communities may well be the most attractive attribute that influences internat organizers to emulate the community model. That this should be so is well explained by the existence of different values and norms for staff members vis-à-vis the residents. This difference may be a major one, as in some internats for juvenile delinquents, or only slightly noticeable, as in many internats for mainstream education. In any case, however, the very purpose of the internat is to help the residents to come to share the value system presented by the staff, which in integrated reclaiming internats represents the values of society. Only in internats where joining the internat is voluntary is there a tendency or at least a strong predisposition, for unified value orientation, as in yeshivas, monasteries, and elite boarding schools. These internats are the models for organizers who ascribe their relative success to their ostensible community-like organization. What is perhaps not fully realized, however, is that their main community-like features derive from what Tonnies (1957) called a "mind community"; as a result, they have fervent supporters in many parts of the broader society. It is not necessarily their egalitarianism, permissiveness, or democratic structure which has made them models of success.

It seems that when a strong unified theme exists, other characteristics of the internat almost automatically adjust themselves to it and become somewhat less important. Belonging and being accepted more become more important that status achievement and upward mobility. Roles are defined, but the quality of role performance is more important than role boundaries and the specific content. To be sure, such an image is usually associated with totality if not totalitarianism, but need it be so? Do we not praise commitment, which is the operationalization of an ideology? Do we not cherish devotion, which is the emotional concomitant of commitment? An ideologically unified, behaviorally committed, and emotionally devoted group of people can, of course, become totalitarian, particularly if deviation is physically restrained and/or severely punished. An internat will be total if exit is impossible or seems to be so, and if there is nothing there to believe in. An internat having a unifying theme along with committed and devoted members may become a "total institution" (in the sense described by Goffman [1961]) if the unifying theme erodes. That is, the framework becomes void of content and the void is filled with proliferated "ideologies," sometimes as many as the number of individual persons residing there.

An example of gradual erosion of the unifying theme can be seen in some of the Israeli youth villages. The prevailing ideology of pre-independence Israel as well as its early post-state period was that of the "chalutz" (pioneer), which manifested itself in a strong tendency toward agricultural work and, in general, toward state-building occupations. This ideology was amply expressed in strong unifying themes in the various youth villages, according to the specific interpretations of the political movement to which each belonged. Since the late 1950s, such ideological orientation have become somewhat eroded in the general society, and also within the internats. Arieli (1980) identified this as a "decrease in ideological commitment" (p. 328). He also noted 5 additional dimensions of change in internats from the 1950s to the 1970s:

a. change from status socialization to role socialization;
b. increase in the importance of instrumental goals;
c. decentralization of the organizational structure;
d. increased role differentiation among staff;
e. increase in centrality of professional affiliation as the focus of an occupational frame of reference for many staff members.

The changes in these six variables mark the transformation of some Israeli internats from a "closed model" in the '50s to an "open model" in the '70s (Arieli, 1980; Kashti et al., 1981). In terms of our discussion, this change indicates a process of change from a community-like organization to a less community-like one, that is, to a more bureaucratic structure. My interpretation of Arieli's observations is that the "decrease in ideological commitment" is the central process and the five additional ones are strategy shifts initiated by the internats to overcome the danger of becoming a totalized framework, devoid of meaningful content. The erosion of the ideological commitment is the least contollable process, yet it is the most influential because it eradicates the sentiments toward ideas which are the ties binding the internat members together. Thus, when "ideology fails," more controllable mechanisms are called for, such as centralized decision-making, instrumentality, and professionalism.

Decision-making. Two major models of decision-making have been proposed for communities. One asserts that decisions which are relevant for the control or governing of the community are made by a "power elite" (Hunter, 1953). The other suggests that decisions are made by negotiation among decentralized, overlapping groups of community members (Dahl, 1961). These two models may complement each other in reclaiming internats. The former works very well when the "power elite" is legitimized by "referent power" (French & Raven, 1960) (the extension of an ideology), or when the elite has "expert power" (the accumulated manifestation of professional expertise and ethos), serving as a unifying theme. If the "power elite" is based on "legitimate (legal) power" or on "coercive power," of course, then authority becomes salient in its threatening connotation, accentuating the totalitarian nature of the internat. The reclaiming source of power, "reward power," seems to be the regulating mechanism of the other four. That is, each power source regulates its activity by allocating rewards and/or punishments. Thus it seems that reward is not a source of power but, rather, a mode of its utilization.

When "referent" or "expert" power is lacking and the internat does not want to rely on "legitimate" or "coercive" power, the negotiating model (agreement among overlapping decentralized groups) of decision-making seems to be useful. The decentralization and, even more, the dispersion of the decision-making process not only fills the gap left by the lacking unifying theme, but it may help to create such a theme. To clarify, the void left by the lack of a unifying theme may lead to the fragmentation of the internat by the way of individual "ideologies," resulting in alienation and ultimately in revolt or apathy. However, when the lack of a unifying theme is accompanied by a dispersed decision-making process, then a new connecting bond is introduced, namely, the communication of conflicts and consents, i.e., negotiation. A dispersed decision-making process exists to the extent to which members of the internat participate in making decisions about their activities. Such participation does not necessarily have to be direct; it can be via representatives, delegates, councils, committees, and other governing bodies, and it can range from symbolic to concrete and from vicarious to direct:

> *Symbolic-vicarious* participation occurs when the internat member is aware that his peers make decisions that concern him. This mode is the most passive, yet requiring that occasions of decision-making are emphasized and publicized. Committee meetings are not secret or even routine but open and talked about.

> *Concrete-vicarious* participation takes place when the internat members see the decision-making process in action. This mode requires members of the internat to be silent witnesses to the debates, negotiations, and voting that take place in the decision-making process.

> *Symbolic-direct* participation occurs when the internat residents elect the various committee members. This mode requires that elections be held often and that members be encouraged to vote.

> *Concrete-direct* participation takes place when the internat member himself is a part of committees engaged in the decision-making.

The actual arrangement of these modes are influenced from within by the size of the internat, the capability levels of residents and staff, and the quality of their interaction. Without knowing these, it is difficult to give a detailed description of the potential participation structure in a specific internat. The principle, however, is that inmates and staff should cooperate in as many regulating bodies of the internat as possible. The outcome of such arrangements is twofold: the structured interaction enhances the assumption of responsibility by the participants for what happens in the setting; and such interaction serves as a control mechanism against the abuse of power either by staff or by inmates. It is important to note that the creation of a committee system can be or can become simply lip-service rather than meaningful "participation" if the committees have no real decision power. It is more useful to exclude certain issues from the discretion of staff-inmate committees *a priori*, than to have them experience that their decisions are not implemented.

In such a structure, a negotiated consensus about the ongoing activity in the internat can develop. This is just a few steps removed from a unifying theme, steps that can be described as compliance, identification, and internalization (Kelman, 1961). A negotiated consensus may yield compliance based on social control and concern with the social outcomes of behavior, requiring surveillance by the governing bodies of the internat. If the attractiveness of the social context grows, however, identification based on cohension may develop. And finally, if the attractiveness does not diminish, then concern with the value congruence of behavior may emerge, leading to value internalization. These stages are parallel with integrated-reclaiming stages of the internat. First, the "Dependent" and "Rule-Dependent" stages requiring close surveillance and compliant behavior. Second, the "Other-Dependent" stage requiring guidance of peers, authority of superiors, and reasonably delimited tasks. Third, the "Inner-Directed" stage, requiring the internalization of the environment's expectations (Wolins & Wozner, 1977).

Developing dispersed decision-making is tedious and time consuming. Obstacles to it are many, on the part of both staff and inmates. Therefore, it is useful that there be a committed core group (staff or, if possible, staff and inmates) to start the process which, once established, can be more easily maintained. Two major conditions are necessary for the establishment and maintenance of such a system, open communication, and graded and specified sanctions.

Communication. Ideally, communication in the internat is open and multi-directional. People communicate both vertically, that is, among the different hierarchical statuses, and horizontally, among their peers. Both directions are important. All members have the opportunity to air their opinions, and information is available to all. There are formal, institutionalized communication channels, such as discussion groups, meetings, newsletters, and bulletin boards, and informal communication is not stifled or disregarded. It is, in fact, encouraged—with the sole qualification that communication about issues of common concern should not be secret.

In practice, these two dimensions, directionality and formalization of communication, are not as clearly actualized as described. Some people may feel secretive about certain issues, and there are always those who believe that they have the right, and even the duty, to censor and regulate the communication flow. Where the principle of open communication exists, however, everyone can (at least in principle) demand the access to information, and the burden of explanation lies with the one who wants to restrict it.

The meaning of open communication is that everyone has the right of access and the right of expression. Conflicts may arise when one is seeking information and another is trying to deny it, or when one wants to express an opinion and another attempts to block it. However, such conflicts can be open to negotiation, which was proposed above as the mechanism for development of a consensus about ongoing activity. When there is initial antagonism and possible conflict of interest between the negotiating parties—such as in internats for delinquents, where conflicting value orientation between reclaimers and the to-be-reclaimed is expected—then special sessions for open communication may be useful.

I have described elsewhere (Wozner, 1965) the use of group discussion in an internat for juvenile delinquents, whereby the boys were encouraged to raise any problem or issue they wished. The purposes were to build trust and teach communication skills, rather than therapy in the traditional sense of the word. A wide range of topics was discussed: experiences in the families, memories prior to their coming to the internat, attitudes toward work and society, sex games and activities, aggression, discrimination, gambling, relationships among themselves, and relationships with staff. Results noticed and attributed to these discussions included an emerging and developing readiness to relate to the issues raised as problems that could be shared, discussed, and often solved, and a gradual decrease in aggressive behavior of the boys among themselves, against the staff, and against the property of the internat. The content of the group discussions was taboo outside the time and place of the discussion itself. During the period when these groups were being conducted, boys began to approach staff members during everyday activities stating "I want to have a discussion with you," or "Let's discuss this problem"; eventually, the formal declaration was dropped and issues were discussed in the normal course of activity. Thus, communication flow was assured. An elaborate description of such a process is provided by Slavson (1954).

The Sanction System. A sanction system can be defined, following Lambert et al. (1970), as the:

> . . . mechanism for maintenance of consensus on value orientation or by which motivation is kept at a level and in the direction necessary for continuing of the operation of the social system toward its ends. (p. 91)

Sanctions (positive or negative) are given because an actor has or has not performed a certain act, or because an actor is to be induced to engage in some activity. Either way, one must be able to define and to declare what acts merit a given sanction and under what circumstances. In other words, the behavior, the sanction, and the contingency have to be defined.

The sanction system obviously concerns both staff and inmates. Measures must be taken to assure that staff members perform their roles and, likewise, to enforce the inmates' activities. The question is whether it is possible to present one system of graded, goal-oriented sanctions appropriate to and accepted by the whole internat. A system of graded sanctions is one in which it is clearly demonstrated that activities functional to goal achievement are positively sanctioned, while dysfunctional ones are negatively sanctioned. To be able to develop such a system, activities must be linked to goal-achievement. That is, the goal itself must be clearly defined and the avenues leading to the goal must be visible.

The importance of a unifying theme and/or the existence of a dispersed decision-making process with an open communication system now became apparent. They all help to crystallize the internat's goals and, thus, present the opportunity to develop a graded sanction system. In truly integrated reclaiming internats, there is one sanction system for staff and inmates, for administrative and reclaiming activities. The main concern of the internat is the behavior of man, whether staff member or inmate. Thus, the contingencies of sanctioning must be specified in all activities for all members of the internat (Wozner, 1979). In addition, the internat's system should consist mainly of positive sanctions, they should be goal-oriented, and negative sanctions should be restricted to limiting interactions which, although aversive, still have the obvious outcome of goal-appropriate behavior.

The sanction system described here differs from the one attributed by Parsons (1968) to the *Gemeinschaft*. The reclaiming strategy of the internat requires that behaviors consistent with the internat's goal as well as behaviors inconsistent with it should be clearly specified. Thus an attitude-specific sanction system will not suffice for a reclaiming strategy which frequently must be detailed and task-oriented.

Sanctions which reinforce or punish a behavior (of a person) may be seen as feedback loops connecting the elements of a social system (Kunkel, 1970; Wozner, 1972; Wolins & Wozner, 1982). In this respect they are "communications" which transpire among the various members of the internat. Not only do they influence the behavior of the others, but they also shape the boundaries of the day-to-day conduct of the members involved. They indicate what behavioral patterns are to be continued and their appropriate circumstances, and they also convey when correction is required. Every communication can be seen as a sanction (positive or negative) and as such it is a feedback loop in the system. An ostensibly sanction-free internat is one in which no communication exists—a functional impossibility.

CONCLUSION

Internats can be organized as communities, albeit they are different in kind from the city and the folk village (Hillery, 1969). The differences pointed out in this paper relate to five major characteristics of the classical *Gemeinschaft*. It is suggested that the community-like internat should have a system of achieved status rather than ascribed status, person-specific rather than task-specific roles, open rather than restricted social and spatial mobility, a unifying theme, and a behavior-specified rather than attitude-specified sanction system. Obviously, the question which presents itself is: Why call it a community when it departs on four characteristics out of five from the classical community model? (see Table 1). The answer is partly sentimental: people seem to like the notion of community and intensely dislike the notion of internat. To be sure, one characteristic, a common value system or, as it is called in this paper, a unifying theme, seems to be central to both the community and the integrated reclaiming internat.

Perhaps this point alone justifies the use of the term, community. There is, of course, more to it than a semantic game. The main force in the integrated reclaiming internat that fuels all reclaiming activities is the unifying theme, from which goal setting, decision-making, the grading of the sanction system, and the social structure originate. When a unifying theme is lacking, such other mechanisms as a dispersed decision-making process, open and multi-directional communication, and a graded sanction system may help to fill the void and lead to the development of a unifying theme. This ostensibly circular description of the variables: unifying theme—decision-making (communication)—graded sanction system—unifying theme, accentuates the systemic nature of the internat, in which the various

Table 1.

Characteristics of Communities and
Integrated-Reclaiming Internats Compared

Characteristic	Community	Integrated-Reclaiming Internat
Status	Ascriptive	Achieved
Role	Task-specific	Person-specific
Mobility	Restricted	Gradually increased
Unifying theme	Exists	Exists
Sanction System	Attitude related	Performance related
Communication	Restricted vertically, open horizontally	Open vertically, open horizontally
Decision-making	Elitist negotiated	Dispersed negotiated

elements (not all discussed here) are in a continuous feedback loop relationship.

The core of the integrated reclaiming internat's organization is that the largest possible number of the members participate maximally in the reclaiming activity. Thus, the issue of whether it is community-like or not is really secondary to the kind, quality, and amount of involvement in the program by all concerned.

REFERENCES

Arieli, M. (1980). The peer group in the residential setting: Some of the features of its informal system. In S. Adiel, Ch. Shalom, & M. Arieli (Eds.), *Fostering deprived youth and residential education.* Tel Aviv: Tcherikover (in Hebrew).

Badley, J. H. (1937). *A schoolmaster's testament: Forty years of educational experience.* Oxford: Basil Blackwell.

Bazeley, E. T. (1948). *Homer Lane and the little commonwealth.* London: G. Allen and Unwin.

Bell, C., & Newby, H. (1971). *Community studies.* London: George Allen and Ltd.

Bentwich, N. (1960). *Ben Shemen: A children's village in Israel.* UNESCO: FICE.

Blau, P. M., Heyderbrand, W. V., & Stauffer, R. E. (1966). The structure of small bureaucracies. *American Sociological Review, 31,* 186.

Dahl, R. (1961). *Who governs?* New Haven: Yale University Press.

Eden (Eisenbach), S. (1951). *The Educational Community.* Tel Aviv: N. Tversky.

Fairweather, G. W. (Ed.). (1964). *Social psychology in treating mental illness: An experimental approach.* New York: Wiley.

Fairweather, A. W., Sanders, W. H., Maynard, H., and Cressler, D. L., with Bleck, D. S. (1969). *Community life for the mentally ill: An alternative to institutional care.* Chicago: Aldine Publishing Co.

French, J. R., & Raven, B. (1960). The bases of social power. In D. Cartwright & A. Zander (Eds.), *Group dynamics.* Evanston, IL: Row, Peterson.

George, R. W., & Stoew, B. L. (1912). *Citizens made and remade* (An interpretation of Significance and Influence of George Junior Republics). Boston and New York. (Cited in Eden, 1951).

Goffman, E. (1961). *Asylums.* New York: Anchor Books.

Golan, S. (1977). *Collective education.* Tel Aviv: Sifriath Hapoalim (in Hebrew).

Hillery, G. A. (1955). Definitions of community: Areas of agreement. *Rural Sociology, 20,* 111-123.

Hillery, G. A. (1969). *Communal organizations.* Chicago: Chicago University Press.

Hunter, F. (1953). *Community power structure.* University of North Carolina Press.

Jones, M. (1953). *The therapeutic community.* New York: Basic Books.

Kashti, Y. (1979). The socializing community: Disadvantaged adolescents in Israeli youth villages. (SEE Monograph Series No. 1) Tel Aviv: Tel Aviv University.

Kashti, Y., Arieli, M., & Wozner, Y. (1981). The Israeli residential setting: Tradition, social context, organization. In Shapira, R., & Adler, C. (Eds.), *Residential education in Israel* (pp. 1-89). Report of the Israeli-American Seminar on out-of-school education. Jerusalem: The Ministry of Education & Culture.

Kelman, H. C. (1961). Process of opinion change. *Public Opinion Quarterly, 25,* 57-78.

Korczak, J. (1967). *Selected works of Janusz Korczak.* Warsaw: Scientific Publications Foreign Cooperation Center of the Central Institute for Scientific, Technical and Economic Information.

Kunkel, J. H. (1970). *Society and economic growth: A behavioral perspective of social change.* New York: Oxford University Press.

Lambert, R., Bullock, R., & Millham, S. (1970). *A manual to the sociology of the school.* London: Weidenfeld & Nicholson.

Lane, H. (1913). *The little commonwealth.* England. (Cited in Eden, 1951).

Makarenko, A. S. (1955). *The road to life: An epic of education.* Moscow: Foreign Languages Publishing House.

Neill, A. S. (1960). *Summerhill: A radical approach to child rearing.* New York: Hart Publishing Co.

Parsons, T. (1956). Suggestions for a sociological approach to the theory of organizations, II. *Administrative Science Quarterly, 1,* 225-239.

Parsons, T. (1968). *The structure of social action* (Vol. II). New York: Free Press.

Porat, R. (1977). *Education in collective communities and in Kibbutzim.* Tel Aviv: Kibbutz Meuchad.

Reinhold, Ch. (Rinott) (1953). *Youth builds its home: Youth Aliyah as an educational movement.* Tel Aviv: Am Oved (in Hebrew).

Reppucci, D. N. (1973). Social psychology of institutional change: General principles for intervention. *American Journal of Community Psychology, 1,* 329-330.

Rinott, Ch. (Reinhold) (1971). Dynamics of Youth Aliyah groups. In M. Wolins & M. Gottesmann (Eds.), *Group care: The educational path of Youth Aliyah.* New York: Gordon & Breach.

Salzman, Ch. G. (1785, 1869). *Noch etwas uber erziehungsanstalt* (Something more on education). Berlin: Richter.

Shalom, Ch. (1980). The role perception of the madrich in residential settings. In S. Adiel, Ch. Shalom, & M. Arieli (Eds.), *Fostering deprived youth and residential education.* (pp. 295-305). Tel Aviv: GOME-Tcherikover (in Hebrew).

Simpson, J. H. (1916). *An experiment in educational self government.* Liverpool: H. Young & Sons. Pp. 105-113.

Slavson, S. R. (1954). *Re-educating the delinquent.* New York: Harper and Brothers.

Super, S. A. (1957). *Alonei Yitzhak: A youth village in Israel.* Jerusalem: International Federation of Children's Communities.

Tonnies, F. (1957). *Community and Society* (C. P. Loomis, transl.). East Lansing: Michigan State Univ. Press.

Watzlawick, P., Weakland, C. E., & Fisch, R. (1974). *Change.* New York: W. W. Norton & Co., Inc.

Wheeler, S. (1966). The structure of formally organized socialization settings. In O. B. Brim, Jr., & S. Wheeler (Eds.). *Socialization after childhood.* New York: John Wiley & Sons, Inc.

Wilensky, H. L. & Lebeaux, C. W. (1958). *Industrial society and social welfare.* New York: Russell Sage.

Wolins, M. (1968). *Young children in institutions: Some additional evidence.* Paper presented at the 45th Annual Meeting of the American Orthopsychiatric Association, Chicago.

Wolins, M., & Gottesmann, M. (1971). (Eds.) *Group care: An Israeli approach, the educational path of Youth Aliyah.* New York: Gordon & Breach.

Wolins, M., & Wozner, Y. (1977). Deinstitutionalization and the benevolent asylum. *Social Service Review, 51,* 604-623.

Wolins, M., & Wozner, Y. (1982). *Revitalizing the residential setting.* San Francisco: Jossey-Bass Publishers.

Wozner, Y. (1965). Meoni: An experiment in the rehabilitation of youth. *Dapim: For social and educational problems.* (Vol. 2, March, pp. 18-25) Jerusalem: Ministry of Social Welfare (in Hebrew).

Wozner, Y. (1972). *Behavior modification and internat care.* Unpublished doctoral dissertation, School of Social Welfare, Univ. of California, Berkeley.

Wozner, Y. (1979). Positive control in institutions. *Residential and Community Child Care Administration, 1,* 187-205.

Community Schools in Israel: The Potential for Integration with Group Care Institutions for Troubled Children and Youth

Ron B. Meier

ABSTRACT. The present article surveys the development of community education and current efforts to adapt this approach to the Israeli educational system. The potential for integration between community schools and group care institutions for children is then assessed. Community education in Israel is found to favor program over process, educational objectives over social problem ones, and is school-based rather than community-based. These characteristics suggest that the community school could act either as an aftercare setting for the troubled child or as a partner with the residential institution in providing an ecologically sound developmental program.

The sheer volume of Jewish immigration to Israel after 1948 and the changing composition of this immigration from almost entirely European to largely Asian and North African (Sephardic) in origin put a great deal of strain on Israeli social institutions, and the systems of residential group care and public education were no exception.

From their inception, Israeli residential care settings were organized as "total youth communities" for the socialization and integration of a largely immigrant population. These institutions were located at a distance from the child's home community and family as a way to make the separation almost total. The residents of these group care settings studied and worked to build a model community

Ron B. Meier is associated with the United Jewish Federation of MetroWest, 60 Glenwood Ave., East Orange, New Jersey 07017. The author would like to acknowledge the cooperation of Yardena Harpaz, Moti Peri, and Yafa Sagiv in completing this research. This article was prepared while the author was at the University of Haifa, Israel.

of peers. The youth were expected to adopt a collective style of life based on their increasing responsibility for the functioning of the community.

The Sephardic families predominant in later waves of immigration did not, however, view the collective principles of Labor Zionism as an ideal, but rather as a threat to their patriarchal family structure and traditional cultural upbringing. Thus, the original system of residential care for children was hard-pressed to adapt to the needs of its changing population.

Nor were Israeli social institutions in general prepared for the high rates of under-education, illiteracy, and poverty among these Oriental Jews. The public education system was originally modeled after the Old German Gymnasia with high standards and a regimen of strict discipline was established (Lipset, 1973), which made it very difficult for the Sephardic child to use the school as a means for social integration and educational advancement. This is reflected in the make-up of the Israeli school population. For example, the percent of pupils whose families came from Asia and Africa was reported to be 61.7% in the 7th grade, 46.1% in the 12th grade, and 14.1% in the university; no similar decline occurred among pupils of European origin (Ministry of Information, 1975). This situation was exacerbated by the official educational policy commitment to equal treatment, which meant that all children, irrespective of their socio-cultural backgrounds and individual attributes, were to be subjected to identical programs in uniform kindergarten and elementary schools (Heller, 1973). Only following riots in Haifa's Wadi Salib in 1959 did the Education Ministry begin to develop special, compensatory programs for the advancement of the Sephardic school population, and implementation was slow in many settings.

In the mid-1970s, the Minister of Education appointed a special committee to investigate the state of Israeli public education. One of its central recommendations was to transform the "traditional" school model to a "community" school approach as a way to establish the school as a primary vehicle for the integration of Israel's numerous ethnic groups (Peled, 1976).

The community school model differs from the traditional school in its commitment to total education rather than education being limited to intellectual training of the child. It departs from the residential group care approach by returning the school to the community and its unique cultural character. It parallels the movement towards community basing in group care, where the links between the agency setting and the family and local community are strengthened as a mechanism for effective socialization, treatment, and education. At the very least, community education and community-based approaches to group care seem to draw on a common ideology which views the community as a central vehicle for child development.

COMMUNITY SCHOOLS/EDUCATION DEFINED

Community education concerns itself with everything affecting the welfare of community residence. In so doing, it "extends the role of . . . education from one of the traditional concepts of teaching children to one of identifying the needs, problems and wants of the community and then assisting in the development of facilities, programs, staff and leadership toward improving the entire community" (Minzey and Olsen, 1969). This in some ways parallels changes occurring in the field of group care for children, where residential care institutions may be seen in new roles in the larger community, as in providing expertise and training for other agencies and direct service to troubled children and their families in their home environments (Beker, 1981). In both community education and in group care, the relationship envisioned between the facility-based program and the community is to be a symbiotic one; that is, the school and group care settings are to draw on the strengths of the community to reach their objectives at the same time as their resources are being utilized to meet community needs.

In the schools, this changing relationship is to be achieved through a transformation of the school itself. The educational program for school-aged children emphasizes community-based elements, i.e., the educational program is made more relevant by moving elements of the community into the classroom and the classroom into the community (Minzey, 1974; Harpaz, 1977). The efficient utilization of all human, physical, and financial resources of the community is stressed through expanded use of school and community facilities (Clark, 1977). Thus, the educational program for school-aged children is complemented by enrichment programs offered after traditional school hours and during vacations. School facilities are opened to children, youth, and adults (including special programs for senior citizens) in the belief that both learning and education are lifelong processes (Clark, 1977). The school is transformed into a center for community activities and problem-solving.

School, community, and family are linked in the hope of creating a better environment for human development and learning. "The philosophy advocates processes and programs to utilize the total community environment and human resources so that the community becomes a dynamic interchange of living-learning experiences for all people" (Decker, 1975). This linkage is also reflected in the leadership of community schools, where community members are extensively involved in educational decision-making. Also, the school takes on a leadership role by coordinating service delivery with the entire network of social agencies and local institutions. Miles (1974) suggests that community education, in fact, provides a context for locality-wide community development.

In the United States, community education as a philosophy of education and model of practice originated in the 1930s (Sandberg and Weaver, 1977). The public school building became the site and vehicle for addressing local community problems through targeted programs. Since that time community education has moved away from problem-centered programming towards the integration of program and process. Services and resources were developed as local needs required through a process of citizen involvement, coordination of local services, and community organization.

Community education in the United Kingdom developed in similar fashion, moving from the "evolutionary" approach of the 1920s to the "revolutionary" one of the 1960s. In the former, community education was school-based and included opening the school to the general community and strengthening home-school ties. In the latter, schools acted as a catalyst for social development and change. The community school's agenda included restructuring of the educational system, community control of schools, reorientation of curricula to local needs and revitalization of the local community (Watson, 1980).

ASSESSING THE IMPACT OF COMMUNITY EDUCATION

Community education has been advocated as a way to address a wide array of societal problems, among them juvenile delinquency, educational disadvantage, public financing of education, school dropouts, race relations, and minority employment (Totten, 1972).

Unfortunately, there have been very few systematic attempts to evaluate the effects in these and other suggested areas (Boyd, 1975). Supporters of the community school model cite success in reducing vandalism, delinquency, probation referrals, truancy, suspensions, and student violence based on their personal observations (Gee, 1974), while critics insist that "programmatically, community education is scarcely reaching beyond that of planned physical activity, formal adult education, and hobby classes" (Van Vorhees, Cwik, and King, 1975). Viewed together, the results of the evaluations completed to date have been decidedly mixed regarding community education's capacity to reach its goals.

The process of community education has developed notably in the direction of the school's role in linking community agencies for service delivery (Sullivan, 1978; Hendrickson and Barber, 1980), but it has consistently failed to bring about the involvement of citizens in program planning and educational policymaking (Watson, 1980; Hendrickson and Barber, 1980). Most community education programs have stressed additional activities for school children and have shown little in the area of development of programming and services for the adult population. Virtually no reliable data are available on the impact of community schools on community problems except in one inconclusive study on school vandalism (Palmer, 1975). Overall, "community education, as a practice, is far from community education as a concept" (Van Vorhees, Cwik and King, 1975).

THE DEVELOPMENT OF COMMUNITY EDUCATION IN ISRAEL

The Israeli public education system is presently engaged in an experiment to try to adapt the community school concept to a somewhat different array of social needs and problems. The idea of community education was introduced in Israel only recently. In 1977, the Ministry of Education and Culture took the lead in establishing a standing committee on community education. A community school pilot project was initiated as a joint effort of the Ministry of Education, the Society for Youth, Sports, and Cultural Centers, and the Israeli Joint Distribution Committee. Between November 1978 and September 1981, eight primary and two secondary schools entered the project for a three-year start-up period. In the fall of 1982, two schools from each of Israel's six school districts were added. Selection of schools for inclusion in the project was based largely on evidence of local initiative taken by the school in stimulating greater involvement of the parents and local community and attempts by the school to use the local environment as a way to enhance the pupils' formal educational experience.

Local involvement was of particular concern given the structure of Israeli school system. Traditionally, the education system in Israel is centralized in the extreme. Schools ". . . are not governed by lay people from the community as in the United States. The concept of a lay board of education does not exist in the Israeli school system'' (Harpaz, 1977). More than this, educational policymaking, decisions regarding school curricula, and all planning, budgeting, and evaluation responsibilities are held by the Ministry of Education at the national level. The impact of such a centralized system has been that parents do not consider it their role to influence the formal educational program that their child receives. In the unusual instances where parents try to influence the local school, they are blocked by the limited authority of the school staff itself in setting policy, revising curricula, or making other educational decisions.

The national steering committee of the community school project reasoned that there would be a greater chance of success in schools that had already strengthened their links to the community. In addition, there was a conscious effort made in the project to prevent over-centralization of authority and to allow the different schools to emphasize very different priorities. Community education was broadly defined as a way to improve the community's quality of life and to strengthen the school's role as a central agent of socialization. Community education was viewed as a process in which the needs, wants, and problems of local residents were translated into programs and activities in the areas of the arts, culture, sports, education, and welfare (Standing Committee on Community Education, 1978).

Smilenski and Baumgarten (1981) surveyed the organizers of the community education project and principals and coordinators in community schools to identify their perceptions of the goals of a community school. Nineteen different goals were mentioned; these can be clustered in four distinct categories:

1. Strengthening Parent-Teacher-Student Relations: developing joint activities between pupils, parents, and teachers; involving

parents and students in school-related subjects; improving the image that teachers hold of the parents and pupils to one of active contributors to the educational process; improving the self-images of the parent and child.

2. Developing Programs and Activities for the Community: initiating cultural activities for community residents; organizing courses for local residents which include professional guidance and advice on educational and family issues; developing supplemental basic educational courses and enrichment activities for those needing them; establishing programs to respond to the needs of groups in the community not normally served by the schools, such as the elderly.

3. Making the School an Agent for Community Development: helping citizens deal with local organizational-bureaucratic problems; integrating the work of different organizations, agencies, and services to prevent overlaps and duplication; improving local services by making them more sensitive and responsive to local needs; giving community residents a greater role in activating local services; aiding residents in organizing to improve living conditions; reducing stereotypes by encouraging greater interaction between community sub-groups; stimulating a positive sense of community identification by citizens.

4. Integrating the Daily School Program with Community Life: making the school curriculum relevant to everyday problems of the family and community; strengthening student activities in the community.

In suggesting community education goals for the Israeli public religious schools, Dagan (1979) incorporates additional concerns: transferring the authority for dealing with area social problems to an autonomous local body with all sectors of the community represented; giving parents real representation on the local school's governing committee; and retraining school principals and teachers for their new roles in the community school.

This comprehensive listing of goals for Israeli community schools should not be taken to mean that there is a consensus about the purposes of community education in Israel. Smilenski and Baumgarten (1981) found significant differences between teachers in different schools and between schools principals and national project directors as to goal priorities. In certain community schools, goals which addressed the needs of pupils and their parents were stressed virtually to the exclusion of the rest of the community. In other schools, great significance was given to reaching the total community. National project organizers and local school personnel differed in their definitions of a model of community education. In contrast, there was almost total agreement on which identified goals not to pursue. The least importance was given to the school's role in conjunction with other agencies, organizations, and authorities in the community. Also, the community school was not seen as a central agent for local community development.

A PRELIMINARY EVALUATION OF ISRAELI COMMUNITY SCHOOLS

In the 1980-81 annual report on the community education project prepared by the Ministry of Education and Culture and the Society for Youth, Sports, and Cultural Centers, major trends in school programming were summarized as being primarily focussed on special interest elective courses offered to school pupils and adults (Standing Committee on Community Education, 1981). Smilenski and Baumgarten (1980) add that the schools often developed one-time special events as well.

The first group of ten community schools began by developing enrichment activities for school pupils and offering courses for adults in the evening. In some cases, this was later supplemented by special cultural activities, field trips, classroom visitation days, and other programs aimed at involving the parents in the community school, but many of the programs just expanded the initial offerings and went no further. The schools that did broaden their programs were characterized by great diversity in focus. The key differences were among programs that emphasized expanding educational opportunities for their students, those that focused on cultural and educational programs for parents and residents, and those that initiated social welfare programs for different populations-in-need.

Our attempt here to evaluate the state of community education in Israel can only be viewed as preliminary, since it is based on limited observations, interviews and, in the work of Smilenski and Baumgarten (1981), questionnaires. One observation shared by the community education committee and by project coordinator Yardena Harpaz is that the community education approach has failed to have any real impact on the regular school program in terms of curriculum or teaching methods. In most cases, the program of formal classroom education and the community education program are largely segregated from each other. In order for community education to impact on the total school environment, it will be necessary to blur the boundary between extra-curricular and curricular activities so that each will contribute to the other.

Nor, at this point, do Israeli community schools seem to be reaching some basic goals regarding the extent and function of public participation in the community education process. The 1980-81 summary report claims that levels of community participation in community school programs have fluctuated tremendously and that many community groups of residents have not been reached at all. One member of the public advisory council in Kiryat Ata estimates that 80% of the adult population attending activities are from the most highly educated, economically affluent portion of the community and would have found similar activities to attend elsewhere.

Results of a small study of parents and other residents who attend activities indicate that a high proportion of participants are satisfied with the programs offered. However, participation by community residents has almost exclusively meant their attendance at programs and activities. The educational staff supports the view that the community school should influence the larger community but has yet to accept the legitimacy of residents "actively influencing what is done in the school in the educational area" (Smilenski and Baumgarten, 1980). Given this lack of commitment, it is not surprising that the public advisory councils seems to be playing a marginal role in decision-making.

APPROACHES TO COMMUNITY EDUCATION

Weaver (1972) suggests that alternative approaches to community education can be classified based on their approach to several key parameters.

Program versus Process

Israeli community schools have clearly favored programs over process. The emphasis has been on initiating activities for school children, their parents and, in some cases, other community residents. In some ways, the community school serves as a community center located on the school grounds. Active community involvement in shaping the community school program is not evident in practice, nor has this been accepted as a necessary and valuable part of community education by the professional school staff. The role of the local community school in coordinating and linking local services seems totally outside the Israeli experience.

School-Based versus Community-Based

Community school programs in Israel have been almost exclusively school-based. In fact, one of the thrusts of the community education approach is to bring the surrounding community of parents and residents into direct contact with the school, its program, and its staff. For this reason, activities are housed in the school building itself whenever possible. None of the ten Israeli schools in the first phase of the project has attempted to disperse its program of activities throughout the community. Yafa Sagiv, principal of a community school in the Haifa area, claims that activities that take place in the schools itself take advantage of the natural connection parents feel with the school but not with other community institutions.

Education-Oriented versus Problem-Oriented

There is little question that community education in Israel has been focussed largely on the goal of educating the child by using the larger community environment. In general, community problems are addressed only as they impact on school-age children, but programs might be developed for the adult community if the home or neighborhood environment was viewed as deficient or inadequate to the developmental needs of the child. The community school has been used as a vehicle to address broader community social problems only in the case of one school where centers for the elderly and for women have been established.

Thus, Israeli community schools have concentrated on developing activities and expanding on the utilization of school and in some cases have attempted to develop a multi-age enrichment program of courses and activities. The role of the community school in bringing about coordinated community services, stimulating community involvement and leadership, and facilitating local community development is not widely evident in practice.

COMMUNITY SCHOOLS AND GROUP CARE
FOR CHILDREN—EVOLVING CONCEPTUAL LINKAGES

Both public schools and group care institutions at one time shared the view that education and/or treatment were best achieved behind closed doors and in a community of professionals and children. Parents and the larger community were excluded to the supposed benefit of the student (Beker, 1981). More recently, the group care field and community education movements have each adopted an ecological approach to education and treatment. Whittaker (1979) stresses that successful treatment of the troubled child is only possible where the total ecology of the child's world, i.e., peer group, school, and family, is addressed. Similarly, the education process within the community school should be based on open exchange with local community institutions and residents.

This changing approach to child and youth development seeks to enhance the role of parents in both the community school and the group care setting by casting them as active partners in the child's education and development. Where parents lack basic educational competencies or specific childrearing skills, the community school should provide educational-development programs for them as a way to better achieve its primary goal of child development. In the group care field there is a growing awareness that residential and day programs for troubled children should function as a family support system rather than treat the child in isolation from his family and home community (Whittaker, 1979). Parent involvement in treatment is being recognized as a key factor in the permanence of therapeutic change (Schopler and Reichler, 1976; Patterson et al., 1975).

In many respects, the Israeli community education experience parallels the development of community-based group care settings both in terms of what they have and have not accomplished and in their attempts to strengthen the relationship between the community and the school or institution. Both have extended their services and programs to serve the adult population, differing only in the degree to which this new clientele has been stressed. Group care agencies have not reached much beyond the children they already serve and their families. Community schools have served groups with no direct link to the student community along with families of children in the schools.

What has been altered in both community education and group

care is the way in which the relationship between the community and its institutions for children is structured in order to reach the program's traditional goals. Neither has revised its basic objectives beyond those of education, socialization, and treatment for its immediate clientele to alternatives such as community organization or coordinating local services.

The group care agency must actively seek the support of community members for its program and residents, particularly when the program is community-based. The community education approach may be of use to the child care agency as a model for enhancing community ties to the institution through an open system in which community residents of all ages become direct beneficiaries of the school program, and, thus, develop a vested interest in its success. More frequently, residential care settings for children and youth try to tap the resources of the community to benefit the child without offering the community a valuable service in return. If they were to open their doors to the community and offer it a range of programs responsive to local needs such as discussion groups, consultations, extension courses, etc., the community would be more likely to accept and support it.

The barrier between the regular classroom and the community education program in schools has a number of important parallels in residential group care institutions. For example, the resident's school program is often entirely divorced from his cottage life experience. This kind of artificial segregation works against the effectiveness of the group care institution by establishing two or more sub-systems each with different expectations, norms, mechanisms of social control, etc. For the resident, continuity is important and such inconsistency can be quite confusing and even destructive (Small and Clarke, 1979), although Eisikovits and Eisikovits (1980) suggest that an autonomous school can provide useful opportunity for reality-testing. The barrier between the regular classroom and the community education program in some schools also finds an analog in the resistance of some institutional personnel to linking the program more closely to the community.

The fields of community education and group care for children are independently moving towards a similar reconceptualization of practice based on the utilization of the total ecology of the child, in which child's parents and home community become more central to the developmental milieu. Further, the once sharp divisions between treatment and education in the group care field and between education and enrichment in the school are being blurred. Both fields are moving toward developmental models of practice. These commonalities are potentially the basis for much greater contact between these two child development systems. The remainder of this paper explores the potential for such networking.

GROUP CARE AND COMMUNITY EDUCATION NETWORKING

In the 1960s and 1970s, many advocated almost total deinstitutionalization of group care for children. Today, it is largely acknowledged that there will continue to be a need for both institutional and community-based care and for a full range of intermediate alternatives (Beker, 1981; Whittaker, 1979; Ainsworth and Fulcher, 1981). The current view is that the needs of troubled children require ". . . an integrated continuum of care that provides a full range of home-based and residential options and contains as easily activated set of linkages between the various service programs and the other major systems in which the child participates" (Whittaker, 1979). This continuum has been conceptualized by Beker (1981) as concentric rings ranging from the least restrictive options at the periphery to the most restrictive ones at the core. The suggestion of an integrated network of child care settings in turn implies greater potential for the community school and residential group care institution to complement one another in providing a total developmental strategy for troubled youth in connection with intake, the in-care, program, and after-care.

Beker (1981) suggests further that community institutions such as the school and group care services are increasingly experiencing a "mutuality of need." Public schools find themselves increasingly required to work with children with a wide range of behavioral, developmental, and environmental problems, and they need the expertise available among residential group care personnel. Residential care settings find it difficult to offer their residents the support systems necessary for successful reintegration within the home community. Such institutions must begin to recognize the importance of bringing their residents into contact with the home community and its major institutions as a bridging vehicle for eventual return to the home setting.

Beker (1981) also offers a possible redefinition of the role of the most specialized settings for the troubled child, e.g., residential centers, as "Centers for Advanced Practice and Research," which could provide expertise, consultation, training, and a research capacity to less restrictive and less specialized settings like the schools. This kind of effort could be especially useful in preparing school staff to deal with difficult or troubled students and providing support and consultation directly to school children with emotional and behavioral problems and their parents.

The community school, for its part, can provide the students and staff of the residential care institution with a balancing, normalizing environment. At certain stages in their developmental program, children who reside in institutional settings can benefit by attending local community schools. This is one way in which children in institutions can learn the skills necessary to function "outside" (Eisikovits and Eisikovits, 1980).

Community schools can also make a contribution to group care agencies by acting as a mediating institution between the community and the residential care setting. This might occur both through the school's efforts to integrate pupils residing in a group setting with those living at home and in attempts to offer services provided by the group care agency to the community through the school's community education program. In so doing, the school would be legitimizing the residential care institution and its residents to the community.

Thus, there is considerable potential for community schools and group care settings to provide their services to both community and institutional residents. When the institutional resident requires a bridge back into the home community as part of a developmental environment, the community school seems appropriate, and when the community resident with special needs requires the expertise of specialized child care professions, the use of day programs in the institution or consultation by its staff seems desirable.

Aftercare Services and the Community School

It is becoming increasingly clear that the outcome for a child or adolescent on his return to his home community from a residential care environment is as much dependent on the support and assistance he receives in the community as on the therapeutic milieu he has left (Allerhand, Weber and Haug, 1966; Cavior, Schmidt and Karacki, 1972; Taylor and Albert, 1973). In the main, such support and assistance comes from one or more of three neighborhood networks: the family, peer group, and the school. Trieschman (1976) notes that group care settings often overlook how crucial school success is to community living.

Community schools programs could make a serious contribution to the existing gap in aftercare services for the child returning to his home environment. The community school generally establishes after-school enrichment programs for the school population, emphasizing activities consistent with what Beker (1981) calls the "growth-enhancement experiences" required for successful child care intervention. In addition, the community school has acknowledged its central role in providing developmental, educational, and social programs to the child's family as a means of contributing to the child's enhanced development.

In community schools in Israel, we have seen the establishment of basic education courses for parents, courses given by school professionals on family issues, and discussion groups comprised of school pupils and their parents on educational concerns and problems. For the troubled child and his family, these kinds of programs provide opportunities for them to view their difficulties and needs in the context of a support group whose members experience similar problems yet within a "normal" environment. Feldman, Wodarski, and Flax (1972) have demonstrated that the mixing of normal and anti-social children in community recreation programs has been quite successful. The community school provides options for such mixing within the child's formal educational, recreational, and enrichment programs as well as in program for the adult population of the community.

Clearly the effective integration of the returning child into the school program and a network of peers can be facilitated through contact between the group care setting and the school. Rothaus and Wolkon (1977) report that the treatment staff of a psychiatric hospital for youth agreed on the importance of such contacts but rarely initiated them, an observation that helps to set the task for all of us. The school needs to be prepared for the child's entry at the same time that the child needs to be prepared for his new setting.

Linking the Israeli Community School with Group Care Institutions

Israeli community schools have emphasized pupil enrichment and parent participation, which are important links to the needs of children residing in a range of group care settings. Group care institutions have developed programs for educating and treating the young person with personal or family problems. Each setting could gain from the services and expertise of the other. For these linkages to be utilized will require the community schools and group care institutions to accept complementary roles in coordinating and integrating services for children. To date, community schools have opened their doors to the community while community-based group care institutions have attempted to open the community to their residents. Overall, neither has sought to work closely with other community or extra-community institutions to develop a system of services for children and youth. This coordinating function is basic to any attempt to bring the community school and group care setting into an effective continuum of care and services for children and youth.

The Israeli community school has not followed the lead of its counterparts in the U.S. and Great Britain in trying to become an agent of social change and community problem-solving. The first community schools in the U.S. were organized to deal with problems of juvenile delinquency. In Israel, community schools were organized as agents of socialization and to improve the child's education through an enhanced learning environment. Problems of economic distress, physical deterioration in the home environment, marital relations, dysfunction in community services, and many others have been viewed as outside the direct cultural/educational/developmental purview of the community school. In general, group care institutions have responded to significant community concerns only as they have been manifested in the individual problems of their residents.

In order to respond more effectively to children with problems, community schools and group care institutions both need to give more attention to the societal problems affecting children. Schools and group care settings will be successful in responding to such problems only as they develop and implement an integrated array of preventive, macro-level interventions, an effort in which they can join forces with much mutual benefit.

REFERENCES

Ainsworth, F., & Fulcher, L. C. (1981). Introduction: Group care for children—concepts and issues. In F. Ainsworth, & L. C. Fulcher (Eds.), *Group care for children: Concept and issues* (pp. 1-15). London: Tavistock Publications.

Allerhand, M. E., Weber, R., & Haugh, M. (1966). *Adaptation and adaptability: The Bellefaire follow-up study*. New York: Child Welfare League of America.

Beker, J. (1981). New roles for group care centers. In F. Ainsworth & L. C. Fulcher (Eds.). *Group care for children: Concept and issues* (pp. 128-147). London: Tavistock Publications.

Boyd, A. (1975). *Evaluation today in community education.* Washington, DC: U.S. Department of HEW, Office of Education.

Cavior, E. C., Schmidt, A., & Karacki, L. (1972). *An evaluation of the Kennedy Youth Center Differential Treatment Program.* Washington, DC: U. S. Bureau of Prisons.

Clark, A. (1977). Community education and its major components. *Journal of Teacher Education, 28,* 5-8.

Dagan, M. (1979). The public religious school as a focal point for community activities. *B'Sadeh Chemed, 23,* 174-180 (in Hebrew).

Decker, E. (1975). Community education: The need for a conceptual framework. *NASSP Bulletin, 59,* 5-15.

Eisikovits, R. A., & Eisikovits, Z. (1980). Detotalizing the institutional experience: The role of the school in the residential treatment of juveniles. *Residential and Community Child Care Administration, 1,* 365-373.

Facts about Israel. (1975). Jerusalem: Ministry of Information.

Feldman, R. A., Wodarski, J. S. & Flax, N. (1972). Treating delinquents in traditional agencies. *Social Work, 17,* 72-77.

Gee, S. (1974). Community schools: Sunnyvale action against delinquency. *Crime Prevention Review, 1,* 25-32,

Harpaz, Y. (1977). *A comparison of typologies of competencies needed for the administrative process of community schools and traditional schools.* Unpublished doctoral dissertation, University of Minnesota.

Heller, C. S. (1973). The emerging consciousness of the ethnic problem among the Jews of Israel. In M. Curtis & M. Chertoff (Eds.). *Israel: Social structure and change.* New Brunswick, New Jersey: Transaction Books.

Hendrickson, L., & Barber, L. (1980). Evaluation and politics: A critical study of a community school program. *Evaluation Review, 4,* 769-787.

Lipset, S. M. (1973). The Israeli dilemma. In M. Curtis & M. Chertoff (Eds.), *Israel: Social structure and change.* New Brunswick, New Jersey: Transaction Books.

Miles, L. S. (1974). Can community development and community education be collaborative? *Journal of the Community Development Society, 5,* 90-97.

Minzey, J. D. (1974). *Community education as a process.* Midland, Michigan: Pendell Publishing Company.

Minzey, J. D., & Olsen, C. R. (1969). *The role of the school in community education.* Midland, Michigan: Pendell Publishing Company.

Palmer, J. L. G. (1975). *A study of the community education program as a deterrent to violence and vandalism in the Alma Community.* Unpublished doctoral dissertation, The University of Michigan.

Patterson, G. R. et al. (1975). *A social learning approach to family intervention.* Eugene, Oregon: Castalia.

Peled, E. (1976). *Report on education in Israel in the 80s.* Jerusalem: Ministry of Education and Culture.

Rothaus, F. D., & Wolkon, G. H. (1977). Continuity of care between the psychiatric hospital and public schools. *Community Mental Health Journal, 13,* 46-53.

Sandberg, J., & Weaver, D. C. (1977). Teachers as community educators training in teacher education colleges. *Journal of Teacher Education, 28,* 9-12.

Schopler, E., & Reichler, R. J. (1976). *Psychopathology and child development: Research and treatment.* New York: Plenum.

Small, R. W., & Clarke, R. B. (1979). Schools as partners in helping. In J. K. Whittaker (Ed.). *Caring for troubled children: Residential treatment in a community context.* San Francisco: Jossey-Bass.

Smilenski, Y., & Baumgarten, D. (1980). *Annual project report: Evaluation of community schools.* Jerusalem: Institute for Developmental Research in Education (in Hebrew).

Smilenski, Y., & Baumgarten, D. (1981). *Community schools: Description and Evaluation.* Jerusalem: The School of Education (in Hebrew).

Standing Committee on Community Education. (1978). *Words of introduction on the broad view of the idea of a community school.* Unpublished report. Jerusalem: Ministry of Education and Culture (in Hebrew).

Standing Committee on Community Education. (1981). *Annual summary report on the community school project, 1980-1981.* Jerusalem: Ministry of Education and Culture (in Hebrew).

Sullivan, K. C. (1978). Measurement of community school development. *Alberta Journal of Educational Research, 24,* 204-212.

Taylor, D. A., & Alpert, S. W. (1973). *Continuity and support following residential treatment.* New York: Child Welfare League of America.

Totten, F. W. (1972). Community education: The feasible reform. *Phi Delta Kappan, 54,* 148-149.

Trieschman, A. E. (1976). The Walker School: An education-based model. *Child Care Quarterly, 5,* 123-135.

Van Vorhees, C., Cwik, J. P., & King, M. J. (1975). Community education has promise. *NASSP Bulletin, 59,* 59-62.

Watson, K. (1980). The growth of community education in the United Kingdom. *International Review of Education, 26,* 273-287.

Weaver, D. C. (1972). A case for theory development in community education. *Phi Delta Kappan, 54,* 154-157.

Whittaker, J. K. (1979). *Caring for troubled children: Residential treatment in a community context.* San Francisco: Jossey-Bass.

III.

Policy Implications

A Policy Analysis of Issues in Residential Care for Children and Youth in Israel: Past, Present, Future

Nachman Sharon

ABSTRACT. The main strength of the child and youth care system in Israel lies at its two extremes: the nuclear family and the child caring institution. For historical and cultural reasons, child caring institutions carry little stigma and enjoy wide public and professional support. In spite of the changes in the populations in the institutions, which currently serve predominantly disadvantaged children and youth, public impressions have not changed radically. Recent trends reflect heavier reliance on community-based services for disadvantaged youth, but efforts to coordinate and improve such services are only beginning.

An American child welfare expert who had recently completed a study tour in Israel has commented that there is no continuum of care for children and youth there, only its two extremes: the family and the institution. It is unclear that other components of this continuum are doing much better in most European countries and in the United States, but the observation holds much truth. The Israeli family in general still seems to be more stable than its U.S. counterpart and, although rates of divorce, separation, and desertion are moving upward, they are still negligible compared to those in America. At the same time, there is heavy reliance on institutions when families fail, even when the failure is not complete. This is almost universally true when dealing with youth over 13 and frequently for younger children as well. Limited changes within the last decade have not altered this basic reality in most situations.

Nachman Sharon, School of Social Work, University of Haifa, Mount Carmel, Haifa 31 999, Israel.

111

Thus, Israel probably has a higher proportion of youth in residential settings than any other country. In a recent year, about 18% of Jewish youth between 13 and 18 were educated in such settings, compared to less than 2% in England and Wales (Lambert et al., 1975). In the United States, the proportion is more difficult to establish because figures are usually given only for populations in correctional and treatment institutions, but there were 238,000 children under 18 in such institutions, less than 1% of the total of this age group, in 1973 (Kadushin, 1974). The 18% in Israel in 1980 was comprised of 37,000 youths in 309 residential settings considered to be alternatives to the ordinary schools (Residential Education in Israel, 1981).

In order to understand the nature of the child welfare system in Israel with its heavy dependence on residential placement, one must follow its evolution within the context of Israeli society and the pre-state Jewish community. Detailed socio-historical analyses of the child welfare and residential system in Israel have appeared elsewhere, including several articles in the current monograph, particularly Weiner (1985), so only a brief overview from a policy perspective follows.

POLICY INFLUENCES INHERITED FROM THE YESHIVA

Although modern Israel is mostly a secular society, the yeshiva has had major influence on its educational thought, philosophy, and policy ranging far beyond the specifics of religious education. The yeshivas today are highly heterogeneous in terms of ideology, political adherence, and curricula, but they share several major assumptions that have set the tone of the residential education movement in general.

First, it is believed that effectively designed residential settings for young people tend to be powerfully conducive to and fostering of cultural and scholastic excellence. All aspects of such settings are geared to enhance elitism. This is in sharp contrast to the tradition of the residential movement in the United States, where such programs are, by and large, designed to be restorative. They tend to view their aim as to restore or otherwise to achieve a minimum or normative level of acceptance. Thus, the ideological and power elite in Israel saw residential education as a status symbol and an avenue for excellence, but the opposite was and is the case in the United States.

Some shifts in population and national priorities have produced limited change in this situation in Israel, but the overall thrust remains unchanged. More residential programs emphasizing scholastic excellence and leadership are available in Israel than anywhere else, with the possible exception of the Soviet Union.

Second, the yeshiva promulgated the idea that individual achievement and group membership cannot only complement but enhance each other. The group was seen as a means to promote social development and adaptation while simultaneously enabling the individual to test out, argue, model, create and, thus, express his uniqueness.

These two assumptions are reflected in such policies as an educational rather than a treatment model of intervention and in the major funding provided for elitist schools such as military academies and secular as well as religious residential high schools. It should be also noted that while residential centers for the neglected and delinquent are under the auspices of the Ministry of Welfare and have a treatment ideology, most residential clients are in institutions under the auspices of the Ministries of Education and Welfare, Youth Aliyah, or specific political sponsorship arising from the conflicts of various groups concerning who will "own" the "heart" of the children—the symbol and embodiment of the future.

POLICY INFLUENCES
FROM THE PRE-STATEHOOD PERIOD

Historical and political circumstances have left their imprint quite irreversibly on residential policies in Israel and have contributed to the complex development of the residential movement. First, with the influx of large numbers of immigrants, many young people needed a physical arrangement to house them. Second, there was an immediate need for acculturation, a way to make these young Jews from a variety of cultures and customs into Israelis as the founding generation understood "Israeliness" at that time. A strong framework of predominant values and ideology was provided to meet this need, while making special arrangements to allow for individual and group idiosyncracies within this framework. A normalizing rather than problemizing ideology was needed not only because it was in line with the predominantly socialist ideology, but also because it was functional to the national agenda to develop the wide range of talents urgently needed by the emerging society. In this context, a massive national vocational program needed to be undertaken as well in order to train young people for various trades and professions.

The fact that such societal needs existed was universally recognized; they might, however, have been met through more community-oriented solutions. The heavy reliance on residential settings instead reflected the preferences of many of the social and educational thinkers from the labor movement, which became the dominant force in the pre-state community. These leaders and educators were profoundly influenced by socialist thought and the German youth movement (Barzel, 1963), and they designed and implemented their own versions of semi-autonomous, collectivistic, residential schools where youth were to be able to assist themselves more freely and and where they could be insulated from the "old world" ideas of the Jewish diaspora that were viewed as anachronistic and dangerous by many Zionist leaders (Shapira, 1966).

Thus, the 1930s and 1940s saw a massive proliferation of residential settings for Jewish youth. The settings varied substantially in their structure, pedagogical methods, and political and cultural orientation, yet they all shared some fundamental common goals that evolved around the creation of a new, homogenized type of Jewish youth who could better contribute to the attainment of national goals. Roughly speaking, the residential settings that dominated the secondary education scene during this period fit three prototypes:

1. The agricultural training schools. Residential settings of this type were established in rural settings, focused on agricultural training and the preparation of skilled cadres for the establishment of future agricultural settlements (Residential Education in Israel, 1981). Strong leadership ability, excellence, and commitment were high priorities. Most of the youth served by these schools came from the more established Jewish community.
2. The youth groups in kibbutzim. These arrangements served mostly immigrant adolescents and some youth from underprivileged backgrounds who were referred by child welfare agencies. Their aim was to work on acculturation and mainstreaming, but many kibbutzim had little real willingness to open themselves to these youngsters (Reinhold, 1953).
3. The youth villages. These villages were established in rural settings, but they emphasized vocational training and acculturation rather than agricultural training.

The second and third types were strongly associated with Youth Aliyah, the organization that served as the primary provider of child and youth services for immigrants on behalf of the Jewish community.

It is possible that by today's standards, many of the pre-state residential institutions would be found lacking. They often substituted idealism, esprit de corps, and strong peer pressures for the systematic delivery of individualized services, but by and large they were successful in achieving the emergent society's goals. They created a legacy that has exerted tremendous influence on the entire educational and child welfare enterprise in Israel and beyond, and much of their present power results from their record of past achievement.

RESIDENTIAL SETTINGS DURING THE FORMATIVE YEARS OF THE STATE

The achievement of independence in 1948 had provided confirmation for the Jewish leadership that their solutions were correct, since they proved effective against all odds and against most experts' advice. This applied to most of the social problems that confronted the new state and, among them, to the problems related to child welfare. Thus, existing policies and operating principles were maintained in spite of the fact that changing patterns of immigration altered the residential population considerably. Youth from other cultures (predominantly Asian and African countries) with uneducated parents and economically limited backgrounds were the new primary target population for residential centers, but little or nothing was done to adopt the old models to new challenges.

The formative years to the 1950s also witnessed the establishment of residential facilities for special populations. Most such programs served juvenile delinquents, the mentally retarded, or the handicapped. (There were almost no facilities for the treatment of emotionally disturbed youth, a type which also became so common in the United States.) The residential programs for special populations were, for the most part, government operated, and many of them bore striking structural similarities to the residential schools for normal youths. In the absence of professionally trained staff and a coherent rehabilitative philosophy, it was hoped that the solutions that had worked so well in the past for normal youth could help to integrate problem youth into the mainstream society. The majority of such special residential facilities were built during the 1950s and early 1960s. Today there are more than 90 in the country (Residential Education in Israel, 1981).

Coinciding with the continuing growth of residential education and socialization efforts, work began in earnest to develop various community-based services for children and families. Day care networks for young children were further developed, and the youth movements made greater but mostly unsuccessful efforts to reach the disadvantaged. Professional expertise was scarce, and the match between the budding community services on the one hand, and Youth Aliyah and other residential agencies with their vast resources and record of achievement on the other, was hardly an equal contest whether the prize was additional client referrals or the expansion of resources. As far as adolescents were concerned, when an assessment was made that a youth needed major support, more often than not the choice was placement in a kibbutz youth group, a youth village, or in a specialized residential facility.

THE LAST TWO DECADES:
THE POPULATION SHIFTS

The current role of the residential facility, that of a provider of services to deprived youth, has emerged in Israel only within the last two decades. It has been a slow, evolutionary process during which the residential facility has lost its dominant role as an educational and socializing setting for the country's elite. Two complementary trends that seemed at first to be unrelated—the gradual withdrawal of middle class youth from residential programs and the massive placement of underprivileged youth in such facilities—have combined to change both the image and the reality of residential services.

Middle class withdrawal was itself the result of at least two primary factors, accelerated by the impact of the changing mix of clientele: the increasing emphasis on educational achievement and occupational mobility, and the return of the nuclear family to its role as the primary socializing agent. These developments both represented a return to more traditional values of Judaism—scholarship and the importance of the family—values that were frequently downgraded during the pre-state era in favor of more radical ones. The value pendulum has now been shifting back from "doers" to "experts," and many of the residential schools—with their rural/agricultural orientation—look increasingly anachronistic in a society that has become more urbanized and technologically sophisticated. At the same time, forces that pushed for separation of youth from their families to enhance socialization have weakened. Established families have tended to become more self-centered and less diffusely idealistic. One result is that they seek to keep adolescents at home and to enroll them in the best possible community secondary schools.

There remain, however, two significant categories of residential programs that have retained their "elite" status. One is comprised of the specialized naval, military, and technical academies, which still attract middle-class youth, especially boys. They maintain high academic standards, and both the military and civilian job markets seek out their graduates. The second exception is comprised of the modern yeshivas that were established in the 1950s and 1960s (Bar-Lev, 1977). It is still quite common, though not essential, for the adolescent children of modern, middle class Orthodox Jews in Israel to attend residential yeshivas. Like the military schools, the yeshivas (and other religious youth villages) have evolved into high quality academic and technological schools, many of which can compete successfully with the best day schools.

INCREASED PLACEMENT OF THE UNDERPRIVILEGED

The large-scale immigration of Jews, especially those from Arab countries, following the establishment of the state precipitated social problems on a scale previously unknown in the country. The strains on the traditional Jewish families from these countries were intense, and serious problems surfaced not only among the first generation immigrants, but among the second and even third as well (Arieli and Kashti, 1977). In the absence of adequate community-based alternatives, especially for adolescents, child welfare organizations turned to the largest reserve of service resources: the residential facilities. They were the preferred choice of child welfare and educational administrators because they had worked in the past and seemed to represent the national ideology. They were also the preferred choice of parents because, unlike community-based substitute care and services, residential education in Israel carried little stigma or implication of parental failure. The connotation was positive—mobility and integration—rather than negative.

From a professional perspective, the placement of these youth in the residential facilities was not seen as confining them in a total, closed system. With their open interaction patterns between youth and staff, these programs were (and frequently still are) regarded as a less restrictive environment than the authoritarian homes from which many of the placed youth came. Finally, Israel's compact geographical dimensions often result in a close proximity between the residential facility in which the youth is placed and his parents' home. Unlike what is frequently the situation in the United States, in these cases the facility may be a home not so far away from home, thus diminishing the feelings and effects of separation.

It should be noted that residential placements were not established as the solution for all or even most youth from non-European backgrounds. Many immigrants from Arab countries have, with increasing success, adopted many of the values and norms of the more established community, and most successful adolescents remain in their own communities to attend local day schools.

THE RESULTING CHANGES

The residential facilities, especially those directly connected with Youth Aliyah, have become more and more homogeneous as a result of these trends. Although the majority of the referred adolescents have not been retarded or disturbed, they have been disadvantaged, and middle-class parents or youth have had little desire to share this kind of experience with such students when secondary school achievement has become so crucial in being able to pursue higher education and career goals. Thus, in 1978, 90% of the children and youth in the Youth Aliyah network came from disadvantaged backgrounds, as did an estimated 80% of those placed in all residential facilities (Residential Education in Israel, 1981).

Some of the residential schools attempted to retain their status, as most systems do when threatened with decline, by changing their objectives, their products, even their clientele. They began to offer more vocational and technological training, entered into agreements with nearby towns for taking in day students, or arranged for technical branches of the armed forces to recruit their graduates. Such arrangements helped mostly to attract more (and more qualified) disadvantaged youth, but they usually did not enable them to retain significant numbers of middle-class youth.

CURRENT STATUS AND FUTURE TRENDS

It is clear that the majority of the population now in residential care in Israel is composed of what has been called interchangeably "youth in trouble," "youth in distress," "youth in need of care," etc. These categories are largely a function of political and professional ideologies and organizational interests, and there is little agreement on who the youth involved are, how many there are of them, and how to handle them. Most Israeli child care personnel seem to agree that "we know whom we mean," and commonly accepted functional aspects of these youths are the ideas that they don't work, they don't study and they are not affiliated meaningfully with any organizational framework. It is also known (although not always acknowledged by all politicians) that the profile of these youth is that there are more boys than girls, ages 12-18, Sephardic (Oriental origin), poor, low socio-economic background, and some sort of behavioral and/or emotional problem. This profile seems close to that of residential care populations in other countries as well.

Another important element in Israel is the advent and proliferation of child and youth services in general and community-based residential care in particular. Until recently most youth services were concentrated in Youth Aliyah and two government ministries (Education and Welfare). Starting with the Israeli Black Panther movement, the resulting social upheaval, and the government's response culminating in the report of the Prime Minister's Commission on Youth, work with distressed youths gained major political and economic significance. Hence a tremendous number of agencies developed a youthwork component or a continuum of youthwork undertakings and attempted to "snatch" clients from others and retain those they had acquired. For example, the army, labor unions, political parties, the Ministry of Construction, the power company, all became new "partners" in the "kid business" (Prime Minister's Committee, 1974).

Little coordination was provided, and many services overlapped and duplicated one another with no information exchange. Referrals were often made based on organizational affiliation rather than client needs. There was no comprehensive policy despite the existence of a centralized system in education and welfare. There were few policy guidelines, and those that existed were seldom implemented on the local level and typically used as a framework to account for what was going on rather than guide it. For example, one could often see three or four workers with seemingly identical functions converging in the juvenile court to testify as to the potential of youngsters to use their unique services and programs.

One result is that proliferation of services, which could lead to coordinated efforts to enrich the possibilities for youth on a continuum of care, led instead to the development of a non-coordinated, highly fragmented youth service field. This is the context in which current day residential care finds itself. Referral to residential centers is often the outcome of the service stream used/available/accessible, rather than differential needs of clients. Also, some child welfare workers believe that it is better to refer youth to residential care just to "protect" them from the chaotic intervention of various social services; unlike in the United States, the residential alternative is still not viewed in Israel as an extreme intervention on the continuum of care. For example, residential care is sometimes used as "preventive placement," that is, youth are placed in "normal" residential education in an effort to avoid the need for placement in other residential facilities designed for disturbed, delinquent, or other problematic adolescents.

Two additional policy trends seem significant in shaping current-day residential care in Israel: recent thinking that investment in after-care, and the use of "half-way" arrangements. While some believe that after-care should be initiated by residential settings and others expect it from community agencies, the concept itself has had a positive effect in trying to organize the efforts of various social agencies working in behalf of children who are about to be released or are in the community. It may be that after-care can be a good conceptual bridge to the development of a client-centered continuum of care. Although half-way arrangements have not become a major social-professional movement, they have influenced both residential facilities and communities toward less dichotomized view of each other and, as Kadushin (1974) and others have predicted, there is currently a little more community in the institutions and a little more institution in the community than before.

It should also be noted that the ideological battle between supporters of institutional placement and supporters of community-based services has been a relatively recent phenomenon. In a pattern common to many technological and professional developments in Israel, the heated debate on this topic that raged in the United States in the 1970s had a delayed impact on the professional community in

Israel. The debate has failed to arouse much passion and zeal, however, at least when one compares it to the ideological and political fanfare that accompanied the closing of institutions in favor of community-based services in the United States. At this point this should come as little surprise to the reader; Israeli residential institutions in Israel have special sentimental value and privileges dating back to the pre-State era. Such special, retroactive privileges carry substantial political weight for many years.

The institutional movement has thus been spared an all-out assault on its philosophical foundations, but criticism has been leveled against certain facilities (especially those for special populations) for not meeting minimum standards. In the absence of sufficient evaluative research, there is not enough information about the effectiveness of several types of institutions that have been serving the disadvantaged populations. There are almost no cost-benefit or cost-effectiveness studies of the kind that were widely utilized at the height of the professional-ideological debate in the U.S. To date, there is limited use of foreign research data as a basis for argument and for decision-making. Yet there is still a feeling among Israeli child welfare professionals that Israeli residential settings have done a better job than many of their American counterparts as depicted in the critical literature. More than community-based services, which seem quite comparable to those utilized in Israel, American residential facilities (as reflected largely in the literature) seem different and alien to the Israeli professional reader whose frame of reference is the Youth Aliyah village.

At this point, it seems that the residential/community-based child care configuration has stabilized in a non-system form, with accepted coexistence but little coordination, mutual utilization, and crossfertilization. This coexistence is reinforced by the political structure of the country. Key ministries and the services under their auspices have been always assigned to certain political parties within a coalition arrangement. Politicians are often reluctant to relinquish a political base by handing over services under their auspices for the sake of coordination. Thus, for example, some youths defined at risk are cared for by gang workers under the auspices of the Youth Division in the Ministry of Education, while other youths who are known as delinquent "belong" to the Youth Division of the Ministry of Labor and Welfare. Similar situations exist in the residential area, of course.

Under these conditions, considerations of professional ideology and judgement become secondary to political exchange. Hence residential care comes to be inseparable from the forces operating in the political arena. Thus, it must be understood that if one wishes to attempt change in the youth care field in Israel, he is into politics. Recognition of this fact, which may also be operative in most other countries as well, may serve the residential field by helping to emphasize that residential care operates in a socio-political context from which it cannot be isolated.

In this light, the residential care system as part of the youth care field should strive to develop communication among and to consolidate the diversified parts of the field, thus fostering progress toward a continuum of care. Thus, the melancholic search for better services can be supplanted by purposive and creative planning, so we can come to terms with the changing social mission of residential care in Israel and, in the light of existing knowledge, develop a future which draws on but does not deify or petrify the glory of the past.

REFERENCES

Arieli, M., & Kashti, Y. (1977). The disadvantaged peer group in the Israeli residential setting. *Jewish Journal of Sociology, 14*(2), 145-155.

Bar-Lev, M. (1977). *The graduates of the Yeshiva high schools in Israel: Between tradition and change.* Ramat Gan, Israel: Bar Ilan University (in Hebrew).

Barzel, H. (1963). *The youth movement: Its development within different countries and in Israel.* Jerusalem: The Zionist Federation (in Hebrew).

Kadushin, A. (1974). Child welfare services. (2nd Ed.). New York: Macmillan Publishing Co., Inc.

Lambert, R., Bullock, R., & Millham, S. (1975). *The chance of a life time? A study of boys and correctional boarding schools in England and Wales.* London: Weidenfeld & Nicholson.

Prime Minister's Committee on Children and Youth. (1974). Report to the Prime Minister. Jerusalem, Israel.

Reinhold (Rinott), C. (1953). *Youth builds its home: Youth Aliyah as an educational movement.* Tel Aviv: Am Oved Publishers (in Hebrew).

Residential Education in Israel. (1981). Jerusalem: The Ministry of Education and Culture.

Shapira, Y. (1966). Education toward defense. In Y. Shapira (Ed.), *Education and settling Tel Aviv.* Culture and Education Publications (in Hebrew). Pp. 219-225.

Weiner, A. (1985). Institutionalizing institutionalization: The historical roots of residential care in Israel. *Child & Youth Services,* 7(3/4), pp. 3-19.

Trends in Residential and Community Care for Dependent Children and Youth in Israel: A Policy Perspective

Eliezer D. Jaffe

ABSTRACT. Policy trends and their underlying ideologies are reviewed for Youth Aliyah, the Ministry of Labor and Social Affairs, and the Ministry of Education and Culture. On this basis, the current status of research and evaluation, differential diagnosis and program assignment, and planning accountability are presented with recommendations for needed policy initiatives.

Institutional placement has been the primary form of care for dependent children and youth in Israel since the establishment of the State and for decades before. The reliance on this form of service stems from a combination of idealogical, economic, philanthropic, and historical factors related to realities of mass immigration and nation-building. Further, once the symbiotic relationship was established between the volunteer organizations which supplied subsidized insitution care and the public welfare departments which contracted and paid for it, this basic pattern became largely self-perpetuating. Institutional placement and group living became the major available tools for re-educative, society-oriented, social-therapy for children, and the empirical success of children's villages and institutions with tens of thousands of children provided increasing momentum and funds for more of the same. Periods of national emergency and large-scale immigration resulted in particularly high rates of placement and expansion of physical plants, staff, and budgets. When peak periods passed, the institutions sought new populations to serve, thus perpetuating themselves, their fundraising apparatus, and their historical, central role in Israeli child welfare. Weiner (1979b) estimated that in 1979 there were approximately 65,000

Eliezer D. Jaffe, Gaza Road, 37, Jerusalem 92383, Israel, is affiliated with The Hebrew University of Jerusalem.

Israeli children living away from home, about 5% of the children in the country, as against a rate of two for 1,000 (.2%) in England and the United States.

It is important to note that not all young people living away from home are placed by welfare agencies, nor are they all dependent or disadvantaged. Israeli society has also been an enthusiastic supporter of residential education for disadvantaged children from large, poor families. In fact, among many sectors of the Israeli population, residential education is identified as a universal, acceptable form of schooling rather than a socially stigmatizing form of child care. Indeed, it would be almost impossible to place so many children today without the consent and cooperation of their parents, and there is research that suggests that some disadvantaged parents view such residential placement as an achievement that offers educational and social rewards to their children (Jaffe, 1970b). The heterogeneity of socio-economic backgrounds of children in various types of residential education also tends to blur the differences between them and between social welfare and purely educational settings.

The impact of policy consideration on the young people involved is indicated on three levels, the first reflecting the ideology, purposes, and practices of each agency. Whether an agency views itself as primarily in the business of education or correction/treatment, for example, has influence on how it operates. A second level is represented by the purchasers of service, normally the Ministry of Education and Culture, the Ministry of Labor and Social Affairs, and Youth Aliyah. Obviously, these agencies can, through their placement decisions, exert strong influence on the shape of child and youth care services. Finally, basic legal mandates—such as those contained in the Compulsory Education Law—have major influence as well. The remainder of the present paper will focus on several policy-related issues as they are reflected in these domains.

INSTITUTIONALIZATION
AND DE-INSTITUTIONALIZATION
AS COMPETING IDEOLOGIES AND TRENDS

New Directions for Youth Aliyah

Traditionally, Youth Aliyah assumed the role of helping Jewish children and youth displaced and often orphaned by the growing tension in Europe around the 1930s and facilitated their care and absorption in the emerging State of Israel. Beginning in the 1950s, however, needs and immigration patterns shifted drastically, with new immigrants coming predominantly from Asia and North Africa, culturally a very different group that might be characterized as "disadvantaged" in the American context. Youth Aliyah served these youngsters as well, only to be faced a decade later with another "wave," this one representing young people born in Israel and living in urban low-income neighborhoods and newly established development towns in isolated areas of the country.

These non-immigrant, disadvantaged children and youth, as was the case with the native-born, urban young people of the 1920s and '30s, were not eligible for the services of Youth Aliyah. Since immigration had fallen off drastically after 1960, however, Youth Aliyah was an organization "all dressed up with no place to go" during this period; it had not reconciled itself to dealing almost entirely with a new, underprivileged, non-immigrant population. These hesitations, both ideological and pedagogical, were criticized by Jaffe (1967; 1983, pp. 234-247) and others who felt that Youth Aliyah should abandon its focus on institutional services to immigrant children and become involved in urban services, child care demonstration work, and child welfare research. Nevertheless, in 1967, Youth Aliyah was still trying in various ways to promote immigration of Jewish youth from the Diaspora to fill its institutions. This group never represented more than about 5 percent of Youth Aliyah's children.

In 1971, Youth Aliyah's vacillation and internal debates over its future were pre-empted by external events. The Israeli "Black Panther" demonstrations in Jerusalem in early 1971 (Cromer, 1976) resulted in the establishment of the Prime Minister's Committee on Disadvantaged Children and Youth to prepare a report on Israel's social problems regarding children and youth. The Sub-Committee on Boarding School Education for Youth Living Away from Home called for rapid expansion of "socializing-educating settings" to deal with the needs of disadvantaged youth. Particular mention was made of the role of Youth Aliyah in the post-Panther era, as can be seen from the following excerpts from the Sub-Committee's report:

> The Committee notes the outstanding contribution of the purposive educational settings and the socializing-educating institutions for disadvantaged children, who lack in their own localities the range of opportunities which the various boarding schools of Israel offer, or who cannot partake of them because

of conditions existing at home. This situation justifies expansion of these opportunities to disadvantaged children . . . It is possible and desirable to enlarge and develop this form of care, despite the fact that the scope of such care in Israel is already quite extensive. It is desirable to develop boarding schools of the purposive and socializing-education types especially for disadvantaged youth. Therefore, it is necessary to encourage organizations such as Youth Aliyah, which is currently interested in developing institutions for disadvantaged youth, and to provide them with the means to exploit the possibilities of this form of education. (Prime Minister's Committee . . . , 1973, pp. 2-3)

These recommendations stemmed from a sense of national emergency regarding the plight of thousands of newly "discovered" disadvantaged youth and coincided with Youth Aliyah's need for a new role in Israeli child welfare. Many of Israel's political leaders, educated in Youth Aliyah or other communal settings, led a popular campaign to increase the scope of residential group care and education in an effort to save more children from the slums and from the problems of overcrowded, urban living. The kibbutzim were also asked to take in more children, and many of them subsequently increased the number of youth groups ("chevrat noar"). In response, Youth Aliyah dramatically took up the challenge and moved into the mainstream of contemporary problems of Israeli urban youth. After a period of gearing up, the Zionist Congress, the Jewish Agency, and Hadassah approved a plan to increase the number of children at Youth Aliyah institutions from 12,000 to 18,000 including a building program for needed additional housing. As a result, more than 50 new residential centers were built, and the number of children at Youth Aliyah facilities increased from 9,000 in 1972 to 19,000 in 1978. By 1980, approximately 67 percent of the children at Youth Aliyah were disadvantaged Israeli-born children, and over 82 percent of all Youth Aliyah children were of Middle-Eastern origin. Within thirty years, the ethnic makeup of the children in care had been almost exactly reversed (Gottesman, 1978; Youth Aliyah Department, 1981).

Along with radical changes in the ethnic, educational, and socio-economic backgrounds of the children in care, the goals of Youth Aliyah also underwent important changes. In the early years the pioneering goals of communal settlement and life on the land were of supreme importance. As a leading Youth Aliyah educator and later Director-General of the Ministry of Education and Culture, put it,

> The (early) goals of Youth Aliyah were to offer (immigrant) youth a home and education, and, later on, accept them as partners in the development of existing agricultural settlements and the founding of new ones. (Rinot, 1960, p. 127)

This orientation was not compatible with the new needs that were reflected in the 1973 report, however, and in the 1970s, vocational training, remedial education, and training for good citizenship became the major goals (Feuerstein & Krasilovsky, 1967, 1969). Twenty-one "youth day centers" were opened, offering vocational and other educational programs in urban areas to 2,275 children living at home. This form of outreach work, undertaken in cooperation with the Ministry of Labor and Social Affairs, was a radical departure from traditional Youth Aliyah residential services.

These population and program changes as well as tightening fiscal constraints combined to stimulate research and evaluation activity at Youth Aliyah, the process and results of which served to further open the organization to new program settings and models. In these ways, community-based options have come to be viewed as viable alternatives for at least some Youth Aliyah clients and have been embraced as Youth Aliyah programs, although the primary commitment to residentially-based services remains. As traditionally a somewhat elite agency in this field, Youth Aliyah has had and retains influence on other service delivery systems beyond its own large numbers of clients served.

Trends at the Ministry of Labor and Social Affairs

While Youth Aliyah serves mostly disadvantaged adolescents, the Ministry of Labor and Social Affairs and the municipal welfare offices serve primarily (but not exclusively) children under age 12 who are dependent, neglected, handicapped, or disadvantaged. These dependent and neglected children constitute approximately 20 percent of all children in institutional care; the others are a mixed group of disadvantaged, immigrant, and upper and middle-income children studying in residential settings. Unlike Youth Aliyah, the Ministry of Labor and Social Affairs has significantly *reduced* the scope of its institution placements in recent years. After a steady increase from 4,721 in 1958 to about 12,000 in 1974, it remained around that level until 1977 and has been dropping since then. In 1979, the total was below 9,000 (State of Israel, 1980, p. 169). What happened to cause this change, especially at a time when Black Panther activities and broader public opinion reflected an apparent need for more placements away from slum neighborhoods?

Three factors seem to have played a role in the Ministry's shift away from institutional care. One was economic; institutional programs, although frequently subsidized from private sources, tended to be significantly more expensive and difficult to finance. Seemingly more important, however, was the increasing conviction at the Ministry of the need to provide community-based services to families and neighborhoods in trouble. The Ministry's response to the problems highlighted by the Black Panthers and the Prime Minister's Report (1973) was to seek more outreach and street-corner social work, more jobs for youth, more school social workers, increased funding for the special needs of low-income families, more community organization work, the establishment of group homes, expansion of foster home programs, and enthusiastic promotion of social and human renewal in slum neighborhoods. The Ministry had taken an ideological turn away from the removal of children and toward community services and the renewal of families. It was acknowledged that it was difficult to guarantee proper supervision and quality care in these settings, and there was increased pressure for expanding foster care rather than relying so heavily on residential placement.

The third factor which led to reduced utilization of institutional care by the Ministry and the municipal social workers was the rejection of institutionalization for babies and very young children. The emotional neglect and sterility of these quasi-hospitals and the overstay rates for children living in them caused many child welfare workers to look upon them as warehouses instead of "baby-homes," as they were called by the women's organizations that operated them. In 1965, there were over 1,000 dependent infants living in nine institutions, with an average of 101 children in each (Child and Youth Department, 1965). Nearly ten years later, in 1974, there were still no less than ten closed institutions for infants, housing 692 children, of whom 90 percent were placed by government welfare workers.

Concern with this situation led to a variety of research projects (e.g., Alt, 1951; Barasch and Jaffe, 1974; Cohen, 1972; Cohen-Raz, 1967; Gewirtz and Gewirtz, 1965; Greenbaum and Landau, 1972; Harpak, Gafil, and Shumlak, 1973; Jaffe, 1983; Rapaport and Marcus, 1976, pp. 181-192; Selai, 1975) that tended to confirm many of the reservations that had emerged regarding the institutionalization of the very young. As early as 1966, the Ministry mandated that the number of beds in "baby homes" be reduced and their efforts be focused on arranging and supporting good foster home care. In 1975, the most prestigious baby home in Israel, where much of the research had been conducted, was closed. In its place came an extensive day care program for over 400 children, a mother-child health center, pre-kindergarten programs, a club for the elderly, and office space for the activities of the sponsoring group in Jerusalem. Another important outcome was the establishment of the "Home For Every Child Society" in 1975.

The closing of this institution and the accumulated research concerning the negative effects of institutional care for the very young resulted in a drastic reduction of the placements by the welfare offices and the Ministry. By 1979, there were only six institutions for infants, each caring for an average of 65 children under five years of age, or a total of 390 children (Goralnik, 1979a, p. 28). At this writing, at least two of these are about to close. Perhaps the most significant outcome of all was a change in policy by the Ministry, reversing its support for institutional care of infants and young children, which helped transform the Ministry from a major buyer of institutional care to an important partner in seeking other alternatives for the problems of small children and their families. This brought events full-circle to the days of Sophia Berger (1928) and Henrietta Szold (1937), who had sought vigorously to provide family care for dependent infants in the 1920s.

The Ministry of Education and Culture: New Partner in Care

Although the Ministry of Education and Culture has been involved in supervising educational programs in institutions and by funding school tuition in residential settings for disadvantaged youth, only since 1975 has it been actively involved in sponsoring residential programs on a large scale. Several residential high schools were established for gifted but disadvantaged students, and the education authorities gradually moved toward increasing concern with issues previously viewed as in the welfare/treatment arena.

In the aftermath of the Black Panther demonstrations and the Prime Minister's Committee on Disadvantaged Children and Youth (1973), the Education Ministry chose group homes as a new field of activity. This avoided the negative aspects of large residential institutions but afforded an opportunity to provide educational and group support for problematic and disadvantaged school children. It provided a closed system of referrals and placement entirely controlled by the Ministry of Education and independent of the Ministry of Labor and Social Affairs.

The Ministry's vehicle for entry into this field was the Recha Freier Institute for Training Land of Israel Youth (Freier, 1939, 1961, 1977). From 1943 to 1975, the Freier program originally pioneered in placing children in kibbutz settings (Jaffe and Lazarowitz, 1970), but, by 1978, three other types of settings were in use as well: children's cottages, children's villages and institutions, and group homes (Cohen, 1972). The Institute's group homes closely followed the pattern developed in many Western countries and by the Ministry of Labor and Social Affairs in Israel.

The children's cottages represented a variation of the classic group home model, involving a series of cottages with either a married couple as cottage "parents" or a housemother and a youth leader ("madrich"). The housemother lived in and took the major role in caring for approximately ten children of homogeneous or, more often, of mixed ages. This model closely resembled that developed by the Austrian S.O.S. Kinderdorf children's villages for dependent children in Europe and other countries (Wachstein, 1963; Dodge, 1972). Although this model found wide support in Israel as a setting for homeless children which combined family life in separate cottages within a familiar youth village framework, some (e.g., Steinitz, 1976, 1981) questioned the importance of mixed age groups, separate kitchens, and the quasi-family living for nine and ten-year old children and criticized the disregard for parental ties. Steinitz claimed that good foster care was better than cottage life in the short run and that smaller, communal, residential-educational settings were better and less expensive in the long run. These arguments were rejected by Cahane (1976), Director of the Recha Freier Institute, who strongly defended this model with its mixed age groups and the availability of a consistent mother figure for young children. Elaborate precautions were taken to keep the maximum number of cottages in one cluster down to four, so as not to create an institutional environment and endanger the intimacy and personalization which constituted the major feature of the cottage setting. Unlike the group homes used by the Ministry of Labor and Social Affairs, most of the cottage settings were owned by the Institute and operated by salaried employees.

As Recha Freier, the founder of the Institute, became older, there was a need to insure future support and expansion. In 1975, the governing body of the Institute was enlarged to include the Ministry of Education and Culture, which took over total funding and operation of the program. The Ministry clearly viewed the Institute as a major vehicle for placing difficult and disadvantaged children referred by school officials (Cahane, 1978b). These developments were greeted with dismay at the Ministry of Labor and Social Affairs which, until then, had been the primary agency for screening and funding the placement of school age children away from home.

After taking responsibility for the Recha Freier program, the Ministry of Education and Culture proceeded to change both the scope and direction of placements. In three years (1977-1979) the Institute's budget rose from 9 to 45 million Israel pounds (Cahane, 1978a, p. 1). The number of group homes increased from two, serving 30 children, in 1975, to eleven settings serving approximately 110 children in 1979. As group homes and cottage settings expanded, foster home placements in kibbutzim declined from over 50 percent of all placements in 1976 to only 23 percent in 1979. Now renamed the Israel Children's Center, the organization is supervised by the Department of Pupil Services of the Ministry, and placement decisions are made by one of the six District Supervisors and the National Supervisor in charge of Family Group Homes of the Ministry of Education. Referrals are made in some cases of neglect and family problems located by the truant officer or school staff.

Mellgren (1978) found that 86 percent of the children placed in 1978 were of Sephardi background, and that almost all were underachievers in school and culturally or emotionally deprived. Two-thirds of the children were males, and siblings were placed together whenever possible. There is an average of ten children ranging in age from three to fifteen years, in the group homes and cottages. At age fifteen, most children are referred to other residential settings. "Parents" in the group homes are often ex-teachers and provide much-needed tutorial help to the children in care. Extra-curricular

activities are encouraged, including membership in youth movements and music and art lessons. Sometimes "madrichim" (youth
leaders) are hired to work with the children, but salaries are low and
working hours inconvenient. Thus, the Ministry of Education has
become deeply involved in providing residential group care service.

The entrance of the Ministry of Education into the child placement field was of great importance due to the political and financial
resources available to it. Within five years, the Ministry placed 59
percent of all the children in group homes or cottages, more than the
Ministry of Labor and Social Affairs and Youth Aliyah combined.
One consequence has been increased competitiveness and friction
with the Ministry of Labor and Social Affairs. Many of the traditional child welfare workers fear that the Education placements are
not professionally evaluated, that possibilities for helping parents
and siblings tend to be ignored by the Education-linked settings, and
the like. It does appear that some of the Ministry of Education programs may, with their residential focus, tend to undercut the deinstitutionalization thrust of Labor and Social Affairs, particularly when
parents who would prefer to have the disturbing child away can play
the two bureaucracies off against each other.

SOME POLICY PERSPECTIVES

Beyond the controversy concerning the preferred forms of substitute child and youth care and the need to develop more effective settings, certain problems and concerns have been identified concerning
the future use of institutional placement and alternative approaches.
These concerns include the need and impact for research and evaluation of various models of care, the significance of differential
diagnosis, and the importance of "master planning" to coordinate
activity in this field.

Research and Evaluation

There has been relatively little systematic study of substitute care
for children and youth in Israel; policy has been based more on
polemics and position papers than on research-informed opinion.
Unfortunately for researchers and for the field and its clientele, the
topic of residential placement has been so controversial and so
ideology-laden that organizations have not always been willing to

provide access to "their" children or their settings. Many are aware of institutional care problems (e.g., overstay, staffing, turnover, emotional neglect) quite well without outside researchers reminding them with numbers and charts, then publicizing it in articles. Where findings do exist, attempts have sometimes been made to hide threatening or unflattering results, but frequently the accumulation of similar results has proceeded until it cannot be ignored, and significant policy changes have followed. The closing of institutions for babies and very young children, described above, is a dramatic example.

More such studies are needed, since they are often the only "voice" that "speaks" for children in care. Thus, empirical research has taught a number of other important lessons in Israel and has eliminated some popular myths:

1. There is evidence that the re-educative peer group in certain residential settings is a socializing agent toward democratic lifestyles and helps establish internalized habits of routine, self-discipline, and decision-making (Jonas, 1964, 1978; Cohen-Raz and Jonas, 1976).
2. We know that persons from different allied professions instinctively favor different types of solutions to family disruption, and that students of social work come to the University with notions of child care that are similar to, and reinforced by, social work faculty (Jaffe, 1970b).
3. Demonstration and experimental research has identified specific factors which determine the type of placement a child will receive, and even how long he will stay there (Jaffe, 1967).
4. Comparative studies of institutionalized children, candidates for institution placement, and "regular" children living at home, have shown better mental health scores for institutional children than for candidates for placement, and the scores of the institution children in general were more similar to those of the regular children (Jaffe, 1969).

Other studies developed and tested research tools for assisting child welfare workers; one utilized a projective test to ascertain children's perceptions of family relationships and found that the strongest feelings and emotional ties which institutional children have are for their siblings (Jaffe, 1977a).

Perhaps more important for influencing the day-to-day life of institutionalized children is the steady flow of studies evaluating the quality and mechanics of institutional care. Jaffe (1977b, 1980), for example, studied the institutional care from the client's point of view and from that of the staff. The latter study found that some staff attitudes (e.g., "saving" children from their parents), high turnover of counselors, poor follow-up, and lack of professional workers in the institution were counter-productive to the goals of institutional care. Lack of continuity and constant breaking of relationships with the children in care has frequently been identified as the most serious problem in institutional placement for children of all ages.

In contrast to research contraindicating institutional placement for young children, Martin Wolins (1974) has assembled evidence of successful group care for adolescents in various countries including the Kinderdorf in Austria, the "djete dom" in Yugoslavia, boarding schools in Russia, Catholic seminaries in the United States, children's institutions in Poland, and the children's villages and youth groups in Israel. Wolins rejects the use of the medical model in assessing group care and the reliance on professionals to influence and shape the group milieu. Instead, he emphasizes the importance of the group itself as a powerful instrument for socialization and as an intervention tool. He notes that collectivist-oriented societies tend to be more supportive of group care, while family-oriented, individualistic societies like the United States have developed negative attitudes about it. He suggests that the forms have managed to provide the kind of continuity and consistency in the group care context that we have indicated above as so crucial.

Thus, despite the relative dearth of research in this area, we have learned much about the necessary ingredients of effective substitute care and how to provide them, work that will need to be expanded and effectively marshalled in support of constructive policy change.

Differential Diagnosis and Program Assignment

Placement decisions, whether for institutional care or other substitute care settings, depend on many factors, including professional diagnoses, availability of placement openings, funding, parental pressures, and ideological and professional biases and beliefs, to name just a few. A study by Jaffe (1979) found that once social workers spell out their criteria for making decisions about child placement and clarify the case history material they use to apply those criteria, a computer can match criteria to case material and reach the same decisions as those of the social workers. But the same study noted that the workers could not always implement what their professional judgement dictated. In these situations, such factors as the unavailability of certain kinds of settings accounted for differences between desired placements and actual placements.

During the 1950s and '60s the availability and acceptance of institutional placement and the lack of alternative programs often led to indiscriminate use of institutions in a situation reminiscent of the adage that if the only tool you have is a hammer, every problem must be viewed as if it were a nail. Differential diagnosis was not widely applied—why bother?—and parental pressures had much influence on placement decisions.

The situation was observed in an experimental study in two municipal welfare offices, where all cases of children approved for institutional placement were re-evaluated by a specially trained team of child welfare workers, who developed differential treatment plans and implemented them over an 18-month period (Jaffe, 1970a). Two welfare offices where no such special reassessments or experimentation took place regarding children scheduled for institutional placement were used as controls. At the end of 18 months there were significant differences in placement rates between experimental and control welfare offices. In the experimental offices, as is reflected in Tables 1 and 2, there was a substantial and

Table 1

Placement Outcomes for Children Referred to

Experimental and Control Welfare Offices,

in Per cents (Jaffe, 1970)

Placement Outcome	Experimental Offices (N = 175)	Control Offices (N = 185)	Totals (N=360)
Institutional Care	39.2	60.8	100.0
Substitute Family Care	52.1	47.9	100.0

Note: Chi^2 = p < .05

Table 2

Placement Goals of Social Workers in

Experimental and Control Welfare Offices (Jaffe, 1970)

Placement Goals	Experimental Offices		Control Offices	
	Percentage	# Cases	Percentage	# Cases
Institution	27.3	(48)	63.2	(117)
Foster Care	23.3	(41)	13.2	(24)
Relatives, Own Home	41.4	(72)	17.9	(33)
Kibbutz	8.0	(14)	5.7	(11)
TOTALS	100.0	(175)	100.0	(185)

Note: $Chi^2 = p < .05$

statistically significant reduction in the percentage of institutional placements, more support for children (and parents) in their own homes, and wider use of foster home care. The reduced utilization of institutionalization was traced to such factors as family-focused versus child-focused social worker orientation, the intensity of family counseling and agency contact with the family, the creativity of the social worker, and efforts to "tailor-make" services in accordance with the specific needs of families observed.

If differential diagnosis is to be reflected in differential program assignments, a range of appropriate program options must be available. In the absence of such options, workers relied heavily on institutional placement, and diagnoses tended to be tailored to placement realities rather than to clients' needs. The study just cited suggests that special workers whose task is explicitly to find and utilize a broader range of alternatives can do so, at best on a limited scale, but this is a costly, idiosyncratic approach that can probably succeed only within rather narrow limits. As policy directions have emerged with legal and bureaucratic sanctions and evolving support in public opinion, however, a broader range of program options has begun to emerge and to be utilized by those responsible for the critical decisions.

Problems of Planning and Accountability

Even before the State of Israel was born, times of crisis produced leadership and services that came to the rescue. The jungle of services that emerged after the 1929 riots was so complex that the Jewish community decided to establish its own Department of Social Work to coordinate the organized social welfare activities. The same problem existed regarding children in need of substitute care. Smilansky (1955), a psychologist and educator, found that many people and agencies were involved in child and youth placement without coordination among them. Each knew how many young people that office had placed and where, but no one had the total picture. This situation led, of course, to duplication and gaps in service, multiple placement of individuals without systematic planning, and other problems.

Almost three decades later, there are still problems that stem from the lack of inter-agency coordination in this field. Two government ministries—Education and Culture, and Labor and Social Affairs—are heavily involved, along with Youth Aliyah, municipal welfare offices, private institutions, and many other agencies. All are operating without any senior, specific national policy guidelines or effort to develop a "master plan" regarding the philosophy and goals of child placement and the development and use of institutional and community program resources. One reason for this is the fact that some of the agencies have grown so large, prestigious, and politically powerful that they cannot be easily controlled. In addition, the desire for the continued infusion of foreign currency and goodwill leads to a reluctance to try to restrict or control agencies with significant foreign linkages. Yet another factor is the inability of one Ministry to openly criticize the program of another or to impinge on its professional "territory," and inter-departmental jealousies militate against the kind of collaboration efforts that could lead to the establishment of broader policy guidelines. Thus, the outcome has been a continuation of the *status quo*, a tacit agreement to live-and-let-live (despite frequent verbal sniping) that serves all the organizational interests concerned but perhaps not the young people and their families who need service or the society as a whole.

Although the implementation of a rational approach to coordination of service to meet client needs more effectively does not seem to be on the horizon, there are a variety of forces at work to help those involved. For example, several groups of child care and social welfare professionals have organized to protect children's rights and to work for reform of harmful institutional practices. ELI, the Israeli Association for Child Protection, was established by interested workers in their fields in 1980 to serve as a watchdog organization for dependent children, and the Israel Association of Social Workers has also become a vocal advocate for reform in child placement practices as institutions, aided by government subsidies, have increasingly added social workers to their staff configurations in recent decades (Appelberg, 1955, 1963; Braver, 1957; Goralnik, 1979a, 1979b; Irus et al., 1964; Jonas, 1964; Rosner, 1965; Spanier, 1963). Although there seems to be little prospect for the development of a lobby of parents of institutionalized children, the Israel Association for the Rights of Large Families ("Zahavi") includes over 20,000 families with at least four children each and has frequently registered resentment at the indiscriminate use of institutionalization to deal with the problems of children from large families in overcrowded housing conditions (Danino, 1978). Finally, more stringent application of its legally-mandated supervisory responsibility by the government can also be a potent instrument to help ameliorate some of the problems.

CONCLUSION

In recent years, a new consensus has begun to emerge among professionals and informed lay people concerned with institutional care for children and youth in Israel. This consensus rejects institutional care for babies and very young children and favors family settings such as foster care and adoptions instead. For ages six to fourteen the recommended types of placement are family foster care, group homes, or cottage-type family-substitute residences. For adolescents, educational and vocational residential institutions and kibbutz youth groups are frequently favored. There is greater sensitivity to the need to explore alternatives to institutional placement, to redefine placement criteria, and to scrutinize institutional philosophies, staffing patterns, and programs so as to promote individualization and personal relationships for children in placement.

Poor agency planning before and during placement, lack of follow-up during placement, excessive caseworker turnover, and neglect of children's parents after placement are the new taboos for child welfare workers. Similar concerns are reflected in many of the reforms and the procedural reorganization introduced by the Ministry of Labor and Social Affairs in the area of family foster care, and they are equally relevant with regard to institutional care since they deal with almost identical problems. Most important is the need to redefine the responsibilities of municipal and district social workers regarding children in placement, and their associated functions, expansion of urban placement settings, and the introduction of paraprofessional and professional manpower on a contractual basis.

With the emergence of these goals, largely a return to an earlier pre-State ideology (Weiner, 1979a) that was submerged as a result of other pressures in recent decades, the direction and the challenge for this field in the years ahead become clear. Greater efforts in research and in coordination seem essential, however, if successful implementation is to follow. Although the pendulum in Israel has swung sharply away from indiscriminate institutional placement to emphasize substitute family settings and community services for children and their families, the rich Israeli heritage of institutional care should not be lost. Perhaps the greater challenge of all lies in the effective, differential use of institutional programs together with other appropriate child and family interventions.

REFERENCES

Alt, H. (1951). Indications for mental health planning for children in Israel. *American Journal of Orthopsychiatry, 21*(1), 105-123.

Appelberg, E. (1955). How and when to tell a child of his adoption. *Megamot, 6,* 148-151 (in Hebrew).

Appelberg, E. (1963). Staff consultation in an Israeli organization for immigrant children. *Social Casework, 44,* 389-396.

Barasch, M., & Jaffe, E. (1974). *Preliminary report of a survey of children resident in the WIZO Baby Home in Jerusalem, Summer, 1973.* Jerusalem: The Hebrew University.

Berger, S. (1928). *Final report (1918-1928) of the Palestine Orphan Committee of the Jewish Joint Distribution Committee.* Jerusalem: Joint Distribution Committee.

Braver, Y. (1957). Individualized care in a children's institution. *SAAD, 1*(5). 153-155 (in Hebrew).

Cahane, J. (1976). The preferred children's home. *SAAD, 20*(5), 67-69 (in Hebrew).

Cahane, J. (1978a). *Report of the (Recha Freier) Institute during 1978.* Jerusalem: Institute for Training Israeli Children (in Hebrew).

Cahane, J. (1978b). On education in the program for training Israeli children. *Society and Welfare, 1,* 498-502.

Child and Youth Department (1965). *Board rates for placement of children outside of their own homes.* Jerusalem: Ministry of Social Welfare (in Hebrew).

Cohen, M. (1972). A survey of young children in institutions who need parents. *SAAD, 16*(16), 91-102 (in Hebrew).

Cohen-Raz, R. (1967). Scalogram analysis of home development sequences of infant behavior as measured by the Bayley Infant Scale of mental development. *Genetic Psychological Monographs, 76*(1), 3-21.

Cohen-Raz, R., & Jonas, B. (1976). A post-residential treatment follow-up of socially and emotionally deviant adolescents in Israel. *Journal of Youth and Adolescence, 5,* 235-250.

Cromer, G. (1976). The Israeli Black Panthers: Fighting for credibility and a cause. *Victimology, 1,* 403-413.

Danino, A. (1978). *The child favored family: Large families in Israel.* Haifa: Zahavi Association for Rights of Large Families.

Dodge, J. (1972). SOS children's villages throughout the world: Substitute or superior service? *Child Welfare, 51,* 344-353.

Feuerstein, R., & Krasilovsky, D. (1967). The treatment group technique. *Israeli Annals of Psychiatry and Related Disciplines, 5*(1), 61-90.

Feuerstein, R., & Krasilovsky, D. (1969). *The meaning of group care within the residential setting for the development of the socioculturally disadvantaged adolescent.* Jerusalem: Youth Aliyah Seminar.

Freier, R. (1939). *Report on social work in Knesset Israel.* Jerusalem: Havaad Haleumi (in Hebrew).

Freier, R. (1961). *Let the children come.* London: Weidenfeld and Nicholson.

Freier, R. (1977). *The institute for training Israeli children.* Jerusalem: Recha Freier Institute (in Hebrew).

Gewirtz, C. H., & Gewirtz, J. (1965). Caretaking settings, background events and behavior differences in four Israeli child rearing environments: Some preliminary trends. In B. M. Foss (Ed.), *Determinants of Infant Behavior.* London: Methuen.

Goralnik, Y. (1979a). *General regulations and board rates for institutions and foster homes, directive 8.17.* Jerusalem: Ministry of Labor and Social Affairs (in Hebrew).

Goralnik, Y. (1979b). *Financial participation in foster care and institution board rates: Employment of social workers, directive 8.18, Appendix 8.* Jerusalem: Ministry of Labor and Social Affairs (in Hebrew).

Gottesman, M. (1978). Youth Aliyah at present. *Society and Welfare, 1,* 484-489 (in Hebrew).

Greenbaum, C., & Landau, R. (1972). Some social responses of infants and mothers in three Israeli child-rearing environments. In F. Monks et al. (Eds.) *Determinants of Behavioral Development.* New York: Academic Press.

Harpak, J., Safil, N., & Shumlak, E. (1973). *The WIZO baby home.* Unpublished senior student thesis, Hebrew University, Jerusalem (in Hebrew).

Irus, R., Orenstein, D., Lifsbitz, E., Fleishman, E., & Shveitzer, Y. (1964). *A definition of the social work function in a closed institution for dependent children: The real and the ideal.* Unpublished senior student thesis, Hebrew University, Jerusalem (in Hebrew).

Jaffe, E. (1967). Correlates of differential placement outcome for dependent children in Israel. *Social Service Review, 41,* 390-401.

Jaffe, E. (1969). Effects of institutionalization on adolescent dependent children. *Child Welfare, 48,* 64-71.

Jaffe, E. (1970a). The impact of experimental services on dependent children referred for institutional care. *Social Work Today, 1*(2), 5-8.

Jaffe, E. (1970b). Professional background and the utilization of institutional care of children as a solution to family crisis. *Human Relations, 23*(1), 15-21.

Jaffe, E. (1977a). Perceptions of family relationships by institutionalized and non-institutionalized dependent children. *Child Psychiatry and Human Development, 8*(2), 81-93.

Jaffe, E. (1977b). Long-term placement of dependent children from the client's point of view. *Mental Health and Society, 3*(2), 300-314.

Jaffe, E. (1979). Computers in child care placement planning. *Social Work, 24,* 380-385.

Jaffe, E. (1980). Institutional care of dependent children from the staff's point of view. *Society and Welfare, 3*(4), 415-427 (in Hebrew).

Jaffe, E. (1983). *Israelis in institutions: Studies in child placement practice and policy.* New York: Gordon and Breach.

Jaffe, E., & Lazarowitz, G. (1970). From outsiders to insiders: Placement of dependent children in the kibbutz. *Applied Social Studies, 2*(1), 27-33.

Jonas, B. (1964). Concerns of the public child welfare institutions: A summary of five years of cooperation between the northern district institutions. *SAAD, 8*(4), 129-131 (in Hebrew).

Jonas, B. (1978). The re-educative institution: A post-residential follow-up. *Society and Welfare, 1,* 464-479 (in Hebrew).

Mellgren, A. (1978). *Family group homes in Israel.* Unpublished seminar paper, University of Minnesota.

Prime Minister's Committee on Disadvantaged Children and Youth. (1973). *Report.* Jerusalem: Prime Minister's Office.

Rapaport, C. & Marcus, J. (1976). *Early child care in Israel.* New York: Gordon & Breach.

Rinot, C. (1960). Youth Aliyah. In M. Smilansky et al. (Eds.) *Child and youth welfare in Israel.* Jerusalem: Henrietta Szold Institute.

Rosner, G. (1965). *Interim report on demonstration in social services in the WIZO Baby Home, Jerusalem.* Jerusalem: Hebrew University.

Selai, Y. (1975). *Long-term institutional care of children.* Jerusalem: Ministry of Social Welfare (in Hebrew).

Smilansky, M. (1955). A survey of services for youth in the transient camps. *Megamot, 6*(2), 153-170 (in Hebrew).

Spanier, Z. (1963). Clinical psychologists in institutions: Treatment methods and organizational requirements. *SAAD, 7*(2), 64-66 (in Hebrew).

State of Israel. (1980). *Budget proposal for the 1980 fiscal year.* Jerusalem: Ministry of Labor and Social Affairs (in Hebrew).

Steinitz, R. (1976). Institution versus foster care: Which is best? *SAAD, 20*(3), 47-50 (in Hebrew).

Steinitz, R., & Olmert, A. (1981). A new attitude towards educational institutions. *Meidaos, 13,* 20-21 (in Hebrew).

Szold, H. (1937). *For children and youth.* Jerusalem: Department of Social Work of the Vaad Haleumi.

Wachstein, S. (1963). An Austrian solution to the problem of child placement. *Child Welfare, 42,* 82-84.

Weiner, A. (1979a). *Differential trends in child placement in the land of Israel, 1918-1945.* Unpublished doctoral dissertation, Hebrew University, Jerusalem.

Weiner, A. (1979b). The child in foster care. *Child Welfare in Israel.* (pp. 303-316). Tel Aviv: Israel Association of Social Workers (in Hebrew).

Wolins, M. (1969). Group care: friend or foe? *Social Work,* 14, 35-53.

Youth Aliyah Department. (1981). *Youth Aliyah student population, 1934-1981.* Jerusalem: Jewish Agency.

Changing Career Patterns
in Israeli Child Care Work

Zvi Eisikovits

ABSTRACT. Changes in career patterns of residential child care workers in Israel during the last fifty years are described and analyzed. Using identity theory and organizational knowledge about careers to generate questions from historical materials, the paper then argues that the present low status of child care work in Israel is related to (1) the changing social mandate of residential care and changing kinds of clients in the system and (2) the lack of fit between existing needs and models of practice.

The wells of creativity lie in time as well as in space; neither science nor art can divorce itself from what has been done in the past: One way or another, the past stays with us constantly. (Nisbet, 1976)

As the child care field struggles with the issue of how to move toward effective professionalism, it would be well to keep Nisbet's observation about the constancy of the past in mind. The models of professional work that are available can best be understood and evaluated within the historical and cultural context in which they developed. The process of choosing appropriate models for the 1980s and beyond can be illuminated by looking systematically at the history of child care work in one rapidly changing culture.

Such an evolutionary approach can highlight several key considerations about the relationship between models of practice in professional child care work and the changing needs of the field including the following:

1. There is a relationship between career patterns of child care workers and the social mandate of the child care institution.

Zvi Eisikovits, School of Social Work, University of Haifa, Mount Carmel, Haifa 31 999, Israel.

2. Efforts to inject pseudo-professional characteristics indiscriminately borrowed from other professions and divorced from the social and historical roots of the field are unlikely to move child care toward effective professionalism.
3. There is a need to identify and evaluate potentially valuable models from the past and resist the modern temptation to use "newism" as our primary criterion. By "newism" (Eaton, 1962) we mean the belief that anything that is "innovative," "experimental," or "new" is automatically superior to the old, the traditional, the familiar.

The purpose of this paper is to clarify the relationship between organizational careers in the child care field and the surrounding historical, social, and cultural contexts. To do this, we will trace the changes in the career patterns of residential child care workers in Israel over the past 50 years. Based on organizational knowledge about career patterns and identity theory, it will be argued that the present low status of residential child care work is related to: (1) the changing social mandate of residential care and the kinds of clients in the system and (2) the lack of fit between existing needs and models of practice.

IDENTITY THEORY AND ORGANIZATIONAL THEORY ABOUT CAREERS

Before turning to the discussion of the last half-century of child care work in Israel, let us briefly examine some underlying concepts related to organizational careers. "Career" can be viewed as a conceptual bridge between the individual and the organization. Following Schein (1971), career in this sense is a set of attributes and experiences of individuals joining, moving through, and leaving organizations. From the organization's perspective, career can be defined as a set of expectations related to a specific social position within the organization, which will influence or determine movement and pace and its timing within the organization.

Looking at organizational career from an interactive perspective, (Blankenship, 1973) means that on the one hand, organizations influence career lines by socializing the individual through such devices as fringe benefits, job responsibilities, power over clients, community sanction, and status within and outside the organization;

on the other side, individuals impact the organization by strategizing about and performing innovative actions. The extent to which the individual influences the organization and the organization influences the individual depends on one's position or stage in the career line and the ways in which the individual's identity interacts with the goals and modus operandi of the organization in a given period.

Identity Theory

Identity is used here in the sense of a person's social position and includes what Robbins (1973) terms identity processes or the interaction strategies by which one establishes and maintains his position in the social order. Following Cooley (1967), Mead (1934) and Goodenough (1963) and drawing heavily on Goffman (1959), this view emphasizes the influence of interaction with others in developing a view of oneself. This means that changes in the person's conception of self need to be validated by social interaction. Hence we speak of identity constituents (Miller, 1963; Robbins, 1973) or identity compact (Wallace, 1967) which is made up of: (a) a person's view of himself or "self-identity," reflecting what he perceives his position to be in regard to others; (b) what others think his social position is or his "public identity"; and (c) what he thinks others believe about him, which is his "social identity." As people go through their careers, they tend to present themselves so that there is a high degree of consonance between these aspects of their identity.

Organizational Theory

In addition to the ways in which the individual's identity influences his movement through the career line, there are also a variety of organizational variables that impact on this process. Organizations can be visualized as a conus cylinder. The three dimensions are: vertical in the hierarchical sense, advancing or declining in rank; radial, toward or away from centrality or the decision-making or power center; and lateral, from one function to another at the same level but in different areas of the organization's activity. For example, a person who starts as a line worker in a child care organization can move up hierarchically, to become a cottage supervisor, area supervisor, perhaps all the way up to the position of director or superintendent. Typically, as a person moves up hierarchically, he also moves centrally toward the power or decision-making locus. On the other hand, it is possible for a veteran line worker to have a central position in the decision making process due to his tenure, relationships with clients, and influence on his peers. An example of lateral movement is for a cottage counselor to become a shop teacher in the center's school.

Each of these dimensions has corresponding boundaries which vary in number, degree of permeability, and types of filtering processes involved. In formal organizations such as schools, hierarchical movement is typically a function of formal education, professional credentialing, experience in the organization, and acceptance by other members. The boundaries in radial movement, i.e., movement toward centrality in the decision-making process, are typically less formal and structured, depending more on political constellations, personal style and influence, and degree of fit between organizational and personal goals. The shop steward of the teachers' union would be an example of a person who may not be moving ahead hierarchically, but is moving toward the power center. Generally, the boundaries of lateral movement such as from being a teacher to be a social worker, or the reverse, are least permeable (Blankenship, 1973).

In the following section, we will apply these key concepts about individual and organizational dimensions of career lines to look at changes in career patterns of Israeli child care workers over the past 50 years and their implications for the present state of the art in child care work in Israel.

CHILD CARE IN ISRAEL IN THE PAST 50 YEARS

The Pre-Statehood Period

The social mandate of the residential care facility in the prestatehood period of the 1930s was two-fold: to educate ideological elites and to inculcate Zionist ideology in new immigrant children arriving primarily from Europe. The long-range goal of the institution was to prepare its residents for agricultural settlement, the embodiment of the Zionist ideology. Since no state-run, centralized educational system existed, political groups or parties tended to have their own educational programs, among which the child care facilities played a crucial role in socializing the young. The educational system had a strong product or outcome orientation (Kashti and Arieli, 1976) in the sense that all efforts were concentrated on the production of an ideal-type, the "chalutz" or pioneer, who at the end of the educational process would settle new territories and become the cultural transmitter of the ideology. No stigma was attached to the client since residential child care was both elitist and universal, i.e., for the brightest as well as the average youth. The holistic view of the resident as an individual and a member of his peer group, rather than only in the role of a client, was the underlying principle of the program.

Programmatically, the child care institution perceived itself as an educational organization in the broadest sense. It stressed that there should be no separation between the institution and the larger community, since education was the mandate of the entire community, not just the residential facility. The program was made up of three components: work, study, and social activities. Special emphasis was placed on the notion that each was of equal significance. A strong value orientation undergirded all three, emphasizing socialism, Zionism, and collectivism. The basic educational unit was the peer group, the nucleus around which all activities in the institution revolved. The program was based on a high degree of self-governance: and young people were involved in making most decisions concerning daily life and long-range plans. There was high consensus about program aims, which went beyond the boundaries of the institution to the long-range goal of settlement. This created a natural continuum of care, with clear-cut expectations.

Identity and Role of the Child Care Worker. The madrich, the child care worker in the institutions of the 1930s, was usually a political activist in one of the ideological youth movements. He or she was expected to have relatively high status within the ideological group in order to be entrusted with a task as important as the education of the future generation for the movement. Implicit in these movements was an ideology of growth and development and democratic youth participation. Typically, the madrich worked in that role for about three years, then moved on to another assignment within the movement. The madrich was the link between the young people and the wider community. The role was a generic one encompassing work with the young people in all three components of the program. Role differentiation was, therefore, limited, with the madrich performing a variety of functions, including teaching, nurturing, and control (Shlasky, 1976).

From an organization perspective, it can be said that being a madrich or child care worker was not just an organizational career in the institution, but rather a stage in an upwardly moving career line within the broader ideological movement. On the hierarchical dimension, the position was a middle-range one, viewed as a springboard and an opportunity to test the leadership ability of a person potentially destined to occupy a top position within the movement. In order to become a madrich, a person had to obtain a certain degree of centrality within the movement. Due to his generic function, the madrich's centrality within the child care institution was undisputed. Having been identified as a person capable of passing on the ideology, the major skill required for the position, he could easily be moved laterally both within the institution and within the movement.

Within the institution, under these conditions, boundaries in all three directions were few in number and highly permeable. The boundaries between the institution and the larger movement were less permeable, and movement through them depended on the level and quality of performance in the role of madrich. In line with the elitist character of the institution, the career line of the madrich was truly meritocratic in this period.

The madrichs of the 1930 perceived themselves as occupying an important social position. To be entrusted with the education of the young meant that one was a person to be emulated. They were also viewed by others as central figures in that these institutions were generally perceived as pivotal for the emergence of the nation (Reinhold, 1953). With high social status, social sanction for his activities, and a great deal of power over the clients, the madrich of the 1930s emerges with a highly coherent identity configuration. This clear, integrated, consistent identity enabled him to perform effectively his job of "guide and mentor" for the clients, and to gain a great deal of satisfaction from it.

Early Statehood

This was the period of mass immigration to the newly established State of Israel from Asia and Africa. The need to absorb a large number of immigrants in a relatively short time impacted dramatically on the social mandate of the child care establishment. The primary goal facing residential child care facilities became the acculturation of large numbers of culturally disadvantaged immigrant children: the making of a new generation of Israelis out of Jews from more than 75 countries. There was now a clear cultural model toward which children were expected to be socialized: the European-born "pioneer" (Kleinberger, 1969).

At this time, the melting pot ideology, which emphasized one ideal type, gave birth to a new social problem—the "culturally deprived." The extent to which a person was culturally deprived was a function of the distance between his particular ethnic and cultural background and the norms set by the pioneers. Another social problem emerged from the effort to implement the melting pot ideology in the "powerful environment" (Wolins, 1969) of the institution. The goal of these institutions was to create "new Israelis" only among the youth population and was not directed toward their parents. Thus, the more successful the acculturation process, the greater the distance that arose between the young person and his family.

On the broad, societal level, two parallel processes occurred: the inclusion of the residential child care movement in the national education system, and a steady process of specialization of institutions by kind of clientele. There were now programs which were academically oriented and those that were vocationally oriented; some were primarily for new immigrants, others for delinquents and some offered para-military education.

On the programmatic level there were several changes as well. The balance between the three program components—education, work, and social activities—shifted according to specialization and client population. For example, the more vocationally oriented institutions emphasized work experience, while programs for the more problematic young people emphasized socialization through various group activities and interactions with staff. In general, there was a strong emphasis on classroom learning at the expense of work and peer group interaction. A major difference now was that the life of the institution revolved around the classroom, not the peer group as it had in the earlier period. With increased specialization of learning activities and the division of labor within the institution, the young person now belonged to many different reference groups simultaneously. For example, he was in class with one group of young people, in recreational activities with another, did chores in the institution with still another group, and perhaps lived with yet another.

Role of the Child Care Worker. As the institutions gradually were divorced from the ideological movements and became part of a state-run centralized educational system, a different type of madrich emerged. In comparison to the madrich of the 1930s the latter was usually younger and less well educated; few had college degrees. Their experience in working with youth came from a variety of settings such as youth movements, the army, and recreation work. As the institutions became increasingly isolated from the community for socialization purposes (the concept of the child care facility as a "powerful environment" was the goal of this separation), the role of the madrich changed. The madrich no longer served as a link between the institution and the broader community, and was left with a rather diffuse role sphere in the institution. With increased specialization and role differentiation within the institution, a variety of professional groups emerged to guide the young clients in various aspects of institutional life. While the stated function of the madrich remained a central-integrative one, the actual role was reduced to helping more professionally trained staff, such as teachers, in performing their tasks. For example, the madrich was expected to help with homework but was not allowed to teach; was expected to make sure the children were on time for their chores, but did not provide on-the-job vocational training; was expected to know what was happening in the peer groups, but was not allowed to do group therapy.

During this period, child care work became an entry level position to a seemingly dead-end career track. From an organizational perspective, there was very little room for hierarchical movement. While it was possible for a beginning child care worker to eventually become a cottage supervisor and even a director, the distance between these steps was so great that few stayed in the occupation long enough to achieve such promotions. To help upgrade their skills, training programs were instituted by the Ministry of Welfare and Education, but these were usually on a para-professional level with low requirements for admission (for example, one did not even need a high school diploma), and hence they did not attract persons with high potential. Talented and upwardly mobile youthworkers typically sought university education in teacher training and/or social work. As an outcome, the best people left the child care field for more formalized and clear-cut career lines in teaching or other human services. With the madrichs functioning more and more as an aide to others to perform their specialized roles, their centrality in the organization depended on performing increasingly pronounced control functions at the expense of nurturance and treatment.

Since there were few tangible rewards for such a low-level, diffused, and difficult role, both the administration and the other professionals in the institution attempted to create the image that the madrich was a "calling," not just a job. This process of image-building was relatively successful. The madrich's self-identity became increasingly anchored in self-sacrifice. He was viewed by others within the institution as a "Jack of all trades." In terms of career movement, others viewed him either as a person with limited ability who was stuck in a dead-end track or as a temporary worker, using his position as a stepping stone to a more professional career. In any case, his public identity was very low. With such a large discrepancy between his personal and public identity, his social identity became blurred. This role diffusion had a negative influence on his working relationships with clients. In a system increasingly geared to specialized treatment, the madrich, left in a role primarily concerned with control, gradually lost his ability to be a guide and model for the young. This, in turn, led to a deterioration of his self-identity.

The Contemporary Scene

A primary emphasis in the national social agenda in recent years is on correcting the mistakes and inequalities that arose out of the rapid accommodation of large waves of immigrants in the 1950s. The failure of the melting pot ideology gradually became recognized, and the model of cultural pluralism has increasingly been adopted by educational policymakers. This, however, could not compensate for the fact that an ever-increasing number of children and youth were lagging behind or dropping out of school, exhibiting a range of behavioral and emotional problems, and making it extremely difficult for their families to cope with their behavior.

The state made increasing appeals to residential facilities to function *in loco parentis*. Overall, the major social mandate placed on institutions is to reduce the social gap between culturally or socially deprived children and the predominantly middle-class European ideal. Consequently, the institutions have become more oriented toward resocialization. Clients are increasingly stigmatized and interchangeably viewed as culturally deprived, socially underprivileged, emotionally and behaviorally disturbed, neglected, mentally ill, suffering from learning disabilities, dropouts, etc.

Two major shifts have occurred in the structure of the institutions to adapt them to these changes in the client population. First, they have moved more and more toward becoming total institutions with a high degree of control and specialization by problem population. There is also a growing degree of isolation from the community stemming from the assumption that such isolation is functional in the resocialization process. Not only is such separation thought to be valuable to the client population, but institutions are also increasingly used to protect the community. This trend is based on the epidemiological or "bad apple" approach, i.e., bad children need to be kept away from good children, to prevent spreading their "disease." Second, the institutions have adopted the medical model in relating to clients. The well-known assumptions of that model include the idea that we can diagnose clients differentially, provide specific and precise rehabilitative cures, and differentially evaluate outcomes. As in the United States and elsewhere, disciplines such as social work, psychology, and psychiatry have, in this context, become influential in defining the ideology and *modus operandi* of the institutions. The normalcy approach underlying the model of the '30s is defined as inappropriate for the populations now being served. At present, youth are *treated, not educated,* with the major aim of treatment generally viewed as personality change.

These changes in the target populations and ideology naturally have led to major program changes. First, the programs now revolve primarily around treatment. In most institutions, there are two competing ideologies: an educational philosophy that stresses development of practical skills, general knowledge, and education for citizenship to enable the young person to become a normal member of society, and the treatment ideology emphasizing the need for personality change as a pre-condition for such an educational program. These competing ideologies are expressed in the day-to-day reality of the institution in the growing influence of treatment personnel in all realms of activity in the institution. For example, in many cases, schooling, work assignments, and recreational activities are all part of the overall treatment plan.

Parallel to the "problemization" of behavior described above, a trend toward the "atomization" of problems has emerged. An individual child is more and more likely to be viewed as the client of various treatment personnel: the special education teacher, the social worker, the psychologist, the psychiatrist, etc. Another aspect of atomization and problemization is that the young resident becomes part of a community of clients under the care of professionals both inside and outside the institution. For example, a social worker working with the child's family may tend to see the young person as part of his caseload. Parallel, the residential social worker is likely to place him also on his caseload. Likewise other professionals such as the drug counsellor or the psychologist may have him on record for specific problems.

It should be noted, however, that the "medical model" has not enjoyed total support in the child care field. Many professionals have become disenchanted with its results and are calling for new approaches. Such "imports" as "deinstitutionalization" and "community-based care" are increasingly being discussed. In the heat of this debate, the fact that Israel once had its own unique brand of community-based care for children has been neglected. Also, as shown by previous Israeli experience in child care, deinstitutionalization does not necessarily mean closing institutions; it may also mean detotalization of institutions from within (Eisikovits and Eisikovits, 1980).

Role of the Child Care Worker. With the growing specialization and problemization in institutions, professionals have increasingly carved out a particular part of the program for their occupational group. Child care workers, however, have largely not participated in the movement toward professionalization, and have been left with the "interstitial" functions not claimed by others. There are no national guidelines spelling out the boundaries and content of child care work; there is no professional association of child care workers; there are no university-based training programs specifically geared for them. This lack of professional status symbols has further solidified the child care worker's role as an aide and a diffuse "Jack-of-all-trades." The result of these trends has been a growing gap in the relative standing of professionals and child care workers in the institution, a trend somewhat contrary to that in recent years in the United States.

Thus, the tendency that began in the 1950s to emphasize control functions at the expense of nurturing activities has accelerated. Possessing neither skills nor formal credentials to compete with others, more established groups of specialists, the madrich became established as "keeper," except in a few settings where such workers were able to carve out a more desirable role by negotiating their particular function within the specific institution in which they work. Since being a generalist can mean everything and nothing at the same time, the madrich was often left at the mercy of internal political struggles and intrigues within institutions. The madrich seldom enjoys status and formal recognition commensurate with the tasks actually performed.

In regard to movement along the three dimensions of career lines in the organization earlier explained, there has been little change since the 1950s. Although the Ministries of Education and Welfare have attempted to create formal career advancement possibilities both in pay and in positions, these have remained primarily at the ideational stage, i.e., not translated into clear-cut policy guidelines. The result is a high drop-out rate among child care personnel and the low level of motivation and preparation typical of persons who stay in the occupation over an extended period (Eisikovits, Chambon, Beker, and Schulman, in press).

CONCLUSIONS

In the foregoing analysis, it has been argued that the social mandate of the child care establishment has shifted from educating ideological and social elites to acculturating the newcomer and resocializing the disadvantaged. Such dramatic shifts have produced massive changes in the programs of institutions, including increasing specialization in and among institutions, growing isolation of institutions from the broader community, and decreasing importance of residential child care on the national agenda. These shifts in the social mandate and programmatic implementation have caused a deterioration in the standing of child care work as an occupation.

Several generalizations can be advanced from this historical survey. First, the analysis demonstrated that the social identity of child care workers is, by and large, a function of the importance of the field's social mandate or place on the national agenda. Secondly, as the social identity of the madrich decreased, there was a parallel deterioration in their personal identity, which in turn impacted on their perceived ability and motivation to manipulate their career line constructively. Third, when institutions fail to adopt appropriate models of practice in the light of changing social needs, certain career lines are displaced or made irrelevant. Movement along these career lines becomes a non-issue when the whole career becomes obsolete.

Under such organizational conditions, professional atrophy of the occupational group sets in. Without a reward structure within the organization, the members of the group will fail to initiate activities leading to innovation and enrichment, which could move the occupational field toward professionalization. Such activities would include the development of a unique knowledge base, skills and techniques, specialized education programs, ethical standards, etc. (Ritzer, 1972; Eisikovits and Beker, 1983).

IMPLICATIONS

If one is to avoid the madrich's predicament, having an occupation that has become obsolete, then it is necessary to broaden the scope of the career line. For example, one could redefine the occupational focus of the madrich as a residential worker, active in a variety of settings with various age groups. Such a model would build sufficient flexibility into the career line to accommodate changing social priorities. One could then easily move, for example, from a line position in a residential child care facility to a middle management position in a residence for the aged.

In a rapidly changing society, one must assume that social priorities will constantly change. Thus, it becomes necessary to design human service organizations such as residential centers with a broader social role rather than to treat comparatively narrow problem populations (Beker, 1981). For example, institutions could be seen not only as providing service for limited numbers of children in need of care outside their home, but also as centers for delivery of a broad range of educational counseling, health and recreational services for the surrounding community. Such a broad-based organizational design would be flexible enough to accommodate changing social priorities.

REFERENCES

Beker, J. (1981). New roles for group care centers. In F. Ainsworth & L. C. Fulcher (Eds.), *Group care for children: Concept and issues* (pp. 128-147). London: Tavistock Publications.

Blankenship, L. R. (1973). Organizational careers: an interactionist perspective. *Sociological Quarterly, 14*(1), 88-98.

Cooley, H. (1967). *Human nature and the social order.* New York: Schocken Books.

Eaton, W. J. (1962). *Walls not a prison make.* Chicago: Charles C. Thomas.

Eisikovits, R., & Eisikovits, Z. (1980). Detotalizing the institutional experience: The role of the school in residential treatment of juveniles. *Residential and Community Child Care Administration, 1*(4), 365-373.

Eisikovits, Z., & Beker, J. (1983). Beyond professionalism: The child and youth care worker as craftsman. *Child Care Quarterly, 12*(2), 93-120.

Eisikovits, Z., Chambon, A., Beker, J., & Schulman, M. (in press). Toward a conceptual schema to assess and foster professionalization in child and youth care work. *Child Care Quarterly,* 15.

Goffman, E. (1959). *The presentation of self in everyday life.* Garden City, N.Y.: Doubleday.

Goodenough, W. H. (1963). *Cooperation in change.* New York: Russell Sage Foundation.

Kashti, Y., & Arieli, M. (Eds.). (1976). *Residential settings: socialization in powerful environments.* Tel Aviv: Daga Books (in Hebrew).

Kleinberger, A. F. (1969). *Society, school and progress in Israel.* New York: Pergamon Press.

Mead, G. H. (1934). *Mind, self and society.* Chicago: University of Chicago Press.

Miller, D. (1963). The study of social relationships: Situation, identity and social interaction. In S. Koch (Ed.), *Psychology: A study of a science.* Vol. 5 (pp. 639-737). New York: McGraw-Hill.

Nisbet, R. (1976). *Sociology as an art form.* New York: Oxford University Press.

Reinhold, C. (1953). *Youth builds its home: Youth Aliyah as an educational movement.* Tel Aviv: Am Oved (in Hebrew).

Ritzer, G. (1972). *Man and his work: Conflict and change.* New York: Meredith Corporation.

Robbins, R. H. (1973). Identity, culture and behavior. In John J. Honigman (Ed.), *The handbook of cultural and social anthropology* (pp. 1199-1222). Chicago: Rand McNally.

Schein, E. H. (1971). The individual, the organization, and the career: A conceptual scheme. *The Journal of Applied Behavioral Science, 7*(4), 401-425.

Schlasky, S. (1976). Changes in the role of the madrich in the residential setting. In Kashti, Y., & Arieli, M. (Eds.), *Residential settings: Socialization in powerful environments* (pp. 144-157). Tel Aviv: Daga Books (in Hebrew).

Wallace, A. F. C. (1967). Identity processes in personality and in culture. In R. Jess & S. Freshbak (Eds.), *Cognition, personality and clinical psychology* (pp. 69-89). San Francisco: Jossey-Bass.

Wolins, M. (1969). Group care: Friend or foe. *Social Work, 14*(1), 37-53.

IV.
Conclusion

Residential Group Care in Community Context: Generalizing the Israeli Experience

Jerome Beker
Zvi Eisikovits

This volume can be viewed as a case study perhaps seeming, at first glance, to have limited generalizability or implications for practice in the field where historical and current conditions differ markedly from those in Israel. This, it seems to us, would be a misconception, and the purpose of what follows is to highlight some broadly useful implications and to point the way toward others, thus also illustrating the importance of national case studies for the field as a whole.

RESIDENTIAL CARE AND NATIONAL DEVELOPMENT

Overall, it seems clear that national development and residential care are intricately interrelated. Residential care is strongest and most relevant when it is able to respond and adapt to the national agenda and even to help shape that agenda in appropriate ways. Thus, when a national priority in Israel was the education and ac-culturation of the elite among immigrants from many countries for societal leadership, and residential programs were designed to meet this need and perceived as successful in doing so, they occupied a central position in the education and human service system and even in the nation as a whole. When residential services and personnel failed to adapt as needs changed, however, this favored position began to erode, and one result is that the resources and influence of the field are greatly diminished (Z. Eisikovits, 1985). In this case,

Jerome Beker, Center for Youth Development and Research, University of Minnesota, St. Paul, MN 55108. Zvi Eisikovits, School of Social Work, University of Haifa, Mount Carmel, Haifa 31 999, Israel.

159

adaptation would have required focusing on children and youth with less social status and influence as well, so some loss in status could have been anticipated in any event, but the social need was great and a successful attempt to meet it would undoubtedly have received recognition. Instead, the field now finds itself forced to deal more narrowly with lower status populations without, in many cases, having developed the will or the skill to do so effectively (Jaffe, 1985).

Creative response to their changing social mandate would, however, have required more of the residential agencies than serving these new, "underclass" populations in residential care more effectively. The "out of sight, out of mind" mentality regarding these groups extends to the settings in which they are placed, a tendency certainly evident in Canada, Europe, and the United States as well as in Israel. Therefore, if residential programs seek and expect to be recognized as playing a significant role on the national scene, they must establish capabilities and roles beyond caring for relatively small numbers of problematic children and youth who tend to be rejected by the rest of society. In Israel until recently, the leadership development function provided this kind of stature. Beker (1981), Carlo (1985), and R. Eisikovits (1985), have suggested some directions that might well be pursued by residential programs in this regard, generally involving enhanced community linkages and broader services provided to communities to help them meet their responsibilities at home for children and youth in difficulty, a role analogous to that of the consultative and community support role of the teaching hospital in the health care sphere.

THE RESIDENTIAL SETTING AND THE COMMUNITY

The social distance between residential programs and the communities they serve seems to vary with changes in the national context. Some residential programs purposefully blur the borders between themselves and the community. Such is the case with traditional child rearing arrangements based on group care within the Kibbutz (Jaffe, 1985; Weiner, 1985). Other residential centers are isolated from the community and seen as "total" or "powerful" environments not to be diluted or contaminated by avoidable community contact (Goffman, 1961; Wolins, 1974). This perspective dominated early residential care in Israel, which was focused on such national goals as implementing a melting-pot ideology of nation-building through the new generation and developing leadership for the country. Reflecting this national agenda, the boundaries separating institutions and communities were clear and relatively impermeable. Whether the residential setting is viewed as a mirror of the community (R. Eisikovits, 1985; Kashti and Arieli, 1985) or as having little in common with it (Wozner, 1985), it seems clear that what is the most desirable relationship between communities and residential centers depends on when and for what purpose.

Thus, if the mandate of the institution is to prepare for life "back home" in the community, as is the case with many delinquency institutions today, such programs seek to establish permeable boundaries and to simulate life in the community as closely as they can. Meier (1985) describes how community agencies can help to bridge the gap in this regard. If, however, the purpose is to prepare people for a different kind of life or different roles than would be available to them outside the residential center, then totality is indicated and interaction and permeability can be viewed as dysfunctional. Wozner (1985) develops some of the basic concepts in which such a perspective might be grounded. It should also be noted that, not only in Israel, one response to the failure of residential settings to achieve their goals has been the idea that they should be more community-oriented and more like the community outside. Based on the Israeli experience, it seems as if this orientation cannot be taken for granted but needs to be examined in the light of the changing purposes and mandates of residential care.

RESIDENTIAL GROUP CARE AND THE FAMILY

Again, expectations of residential settings in Israel shifted with changing national attitudes and purposes concerning such issues as relative responsibilities of the family and the state towards the child and the function of the family in relation to that of the residential setting. When the residential center was believed to be a primary agent in nation-building and the family was viewed as a regressive institution standing in the way of this process, residential care made every effort to isolate children from their families, both physically and psychologically. This was true both in the Kibbutz and in the Youth Aliyah programs serving primarily urban children and youth. More recently, with the shifts we have observed in the populations served and in the social mandate of the institution, views on relationships with families have also shifted. Maintaining continuous contact with families and involving parents as much as possible is now viewed as part of the "reclaiming" process (Laufer, 1985).

These changing views regarding the importance of the family were also associated with broader societal changes that resulted in parents being expected to assume greater responsibility for the development and the behavior of their children. Thus, when residential care was charged with educating the elite and other nation-building functions (Sharon, 1985; Jaffe, 1985), parents were excluded; when the focus shifted to emphasize rehabilitation, correction, and reintegration, parents were not only included but were held responsible. Incidentally, it will be important to note the impact of the widening provision of day care services for the children of working parents on the expectations held of parents and community services.

THE GROUP AND THE FAMILY IN GROUP CARE

An additional, related trend can be explored on the basis of the Israeli experience: the changing role of the group in group care. The importance of the group as the basic living, learning, and treatment unit seems to be inversely related to the importance of the family. Thus, the group was the basic program unit in early residential care, when the family was viewed as unimportant; later, the group tended to be neglected as emphasis was increasingly placed on family ties and involvement. The implementation of the continuum of care idea in Israel, as elsewhere, tends to emphasize the role of the family and gives less salience to group living phenomena.

THE IMPACT ON GROUP CARE PERSONNEL

Concomitant with the shifting emphasis in residential care toward amelioration of what are viewed as social and personal deficits (e.g., rehabilitation, re-socialization, and re-integration), residential care workers are increasingly expected to be specialized professionals rather than more eclectic substitute parents, role models, and leaders. This trend toward professionalization is associated with returning the parental function to the parents and with new responsibilities for the worker in making this transition. Insofar as possible, intervention is viewed in the family context, and success is defined largely in terms of the goal of returning the child to the family. It seems clear that trends toward professionalization and toward involvement with families are directly related.

The shift from generalist to specialist is only one aspect of change in the role of the child and youth care worker. Formerly viewed as idealogues who relied heavily on personal charisma and role modelling, such workers are now expected to use knowledge and themselves consciously in a wide variety of situations both within and beyond the group care context. Increasingly, they are pressed to respond from a developmental or treatment perspective rather than a political or custodial one, and the career line as well as the group care setting itself tends to become a dead-end where the objective for staff and residents alike is to get better and get out—and to launch the successful worker on a broader career in political leadership and societal development—rather than to mirror and model a social ideal (Z. Eisikovits, 1985).

In general it seems clear than when residential child care has a more significant and prestigeful social mandate, so does the worker. When the field stagnates and career patterns do not take account of changing social needs and opportunities, one can expect the status of child care workers to deteriorate and their significance and influence in society to weaken. In this connection, it might be suggested that the tendency for many child and youth care workers may be to operate more as specialized residential treatment professionals when what the field and the society need are workers with greater competence in the skills of community organization both within and beyond the institution, as was the case when the field occupied a more prominent position. In this context, a significant question arises as to the effects of the status and orientation of group care personnel on the young people in group care programs.

THE RESIDENTIAL CENTER AND ITS CLIENTELE

It has become clear by now that decisions about who will be placed in a residential setting are not simply a function of the needs of the young people involved and their parents. Such factors as which professional sees a child first and even simple availability of beds impact heavily on such decisions (e.g., Krisberg and Schwartz, 1983). The Israeli experience demonstrates that the prevailing social agenda for residential care and even political affiliations of the family may be important factors. Thus, both the intake and the impact of such programs differ if they are viewed as preparing the elite, enculturating an immigrant population, or rehabilitating problematic youth. Particularly in the first two categories, ideologically-based political parties in Israel have had a stake in residential programs as well, often expressed through competition for the "best" candidates to fill their proportional intake quotas (Weiner, 1985; Jaffe, 1985), not unlike the competition that occurs elsewhere to "cream" the best (least troublesome) candidates among available applicants. Thus, simply knowing the characteristics of the population is not enough; it is important to understand the intricate, dynamic interplay among such subtle social forces as a basis for effective work in residential care and to enhance the development of the field.

Internally, as has been noted, the residential program may be viewed as a mirror of the community, undoubtedly with some distortions, or as a total departure from it. It appears that this choice should be a function of the desired outcome: if the objective is to create citizens who will "fit in," then the institution should be community-like; if the child is expected to change so as to be different from the broader community, then the differences between the community and the institution should be stressed.

We generally think of "good" institutions for children and youth as geared and responsive to children's needs in the present and as helping to prepare them for future roles in society; therefore, we expect them to be child-centered. The Israeli experience highlights, perhaps, that what children "need" is socially, politically, and culturally prescribed; such "social prescriptions" respond to factors other than what children actually need from a developmental perspective. Even in a child-centered society like Israel's, it would be naive to try to understand the community implications of residential programs or any other elements of group care for children and youth outside this complex socio-political context. To integrate these often conflicting streams in a professionally responsible manner is a fundamental intellectual and practical challenge for all of us in our day-to-day work in the field.

REFERENCES

Beker, J. (1981). New roles for group care centers. In F. Ainsworth & L. C. Fulcher (Eds.), *Group care for children: concept and issues* (pp. 128-147). London: Tavistock Publications.

Carlo, P. (1985). The children's residential center as a living laboratory for family members:

A review of the literature and its implications for practice. *Child Care Quarterly, 14*(3), in press.

Eisikovits, R. A. (1985). Children's institutions in Israel as mirrors of social and cultural change. *Child & Youth Services, 7*(3/4), pp. 21-29.

Eisikovits, Z. (1985). Changing career patterns in Israeli child care work. *Child & Youth Services, 7*(3/4), pp. 143-156.

Goffman, E. (1961). *Asylums.* New York: Doubleday.

Jaffe, E. D. (1985). Trends in residential and community care for dependent children and youth in Israel: A policy perspective. *Child & Youth Services, 7*(3/4), pp. 123-141.

Kashti, Y., & Arieli, M. (1985). Social conditions and pupils' responses in Israeli residential schools. *Child & Youth Services, 7*(3/4), pp. 51-70.

Krisberg, B., & Schwartz, I. (1983). Rethinking juvenile justice. *Crime & Delinquency, 29,* 333-364.

Laufer, Z. (1985). Institutional placement: An interim stage or an end in itself? The role of parents in the continuum of care. *Child & Youth Services, 7*(3/4), pp. 33-50.

Meier, R. B. (1985). Community schools in Israel: The potential for integration with group care institutions for troubled children and youth. *Child & Youth Services, 7*(3/4), pp. 91-108.

Sharon, N. (1985). A policy analysis of issues in residential care for children and youth in Israel: Past, present, future. *Child & Youth Services, 7*(3/4), pp. 111-122.

Weiner. A. (1985). Institutionalizing institutionalization: The historical roots of residential care in Israel. *Child & Youth Services, 7*(3/4), pp. 3-19.

Wolins, M. (Ed.) (1974). *Successful group care: Explorations in the powerful environment.* Chicago: Aldine.

Wozner, Y. (1985). Institution as community. *Child & Youth Services, 7*(3/4), pp. 71-89.

Index